The Complete Ketogenic Diet, Mediterranean Diet, Instant Pot Recipe Cookbook & Intermittent Fasting

Table of Contents

Ketogenic Diet for Beginners: 3

Mediterranean Diet 30

Instant Pot Recipes Cookbook 58

The Complete Guide to Intermittent Fasting 91

Ketogenic Diet for Beginners:

Lose a Lot of Weight Fast Using Your Body's Natural Processes

Charlie Mason

© Copyright 2017 by Charlie Mason- All rights reserved.

The following eBook is reproduced below with the goal of providing information that is as accurate and reliable as possible. Regardless, purchasing this eBook can be seen as consent to the fact that both the publisher and the author of this book are in no way experts on the topics discussed within and that any recommendations or suggestions that are made herein are for entertainment purposes only. Professionals should be consulted as needed prior to undertaking any of the action endorsed herein. This declaration is deemed fair and valid by both the American Bar Association and the Committee of Publishers Association and is legally binding throughout the United States. Furthermore, the transmission, duplication or reproduction of any of the following work including specific information will be considered an illegal act irrespective of if it is done electronically or in print. This extends to creating a secondary or tertiary copy of the work or a recorded copy and is only allowed with express written consent of the Publisher. All additional right reserved.

The information in the following pages is broadly considered to be a truthful and accurate account of facts and as such any inattention, use or misuse of the information in question by the reader will render any resulting actions solely under their purview. There are no scenarios in which the publisher or the original author of this work can be in any fashion deemed liable for any hardship or damages that may befall them after undertaking information described herein.

Additionally, the information in the following pages is intended only for informational purposes and should thus be thought of as universal. As befitting its nature, it is presented without assurance regarding its prolonged validity or interim quality. Trademarks that are mentioned are done without written consent and can in no way be considered an endorsement from the trademark holder.

Introduction

Congratulations on getting this book and thank you for doing so. The following chapters will discuss how to use the ketogenic diet to achieve your weight loss goals.

There are plenty of books on this subject on the market, thanks again for choosing this one! Every effort was made to ensure it is full of as much useful information as possible, please enjoy!

BONUS:

As a way of saying thank you for purchasing my book, please use your link below to claim your 3 FREE Cookbooks on Health, Fitness & Dieting Instantly

https://bit.ly/2OazEZu

You can also share your link with your friends and families whom you think that can benefit from the cookbooks or you can forward them the link as a gift!

At the end of every bundle can you copy and paste this:

** Remember to use your link to claim your 3 FREE Cookbooks on Health, Fitness & Dieting Instantly

https://bit.ly/2OazEZu

CHAPTER 1

How Ketosis Can Benefit You

If I told you that your body had a natural system for burning fat that you simply weren't utilizing, would you believe me? Most people wouldn't. However, more and more people are coming around to this wonderful diet in what I like to call the low-carb revolution.

The purpose of the ketogenic diet is to retrain your body to run on better fuel. Rather than glucose, your body will learn to run on fat for fuel. Eating this way will place your body in a position wherein it primarily uses fat, rather than sugar for energy.

However, the ketogenic diet is focused on one key concept: *ketosis*. *Ketosis* is, to simply say, an alternative way that the body can burn fuel. When one is in a state of *ketosis*, then they are burning what are called *ketones* for energy, instead of *carbohydrates* like usual. Ketones can be generated from both the body's fat deposits and stores, as well as from ingested fat. This leads us to the first way that ketosis can benefit you: you'll be *less hungry*. We'll talk more about the simple mechanics of weight loss either, but for right now, just understand this: fats burn *slower* than carbs do, which means that you'll be a lot less hungry a lot less often.

Moreover, when you're eating *less* energy than your body is taking out, your body takes energy *directly* from your natural fat stores without any sort of conversion process, meaning that you'll shed pounds like crazy.

When you eat a diet that is heavy in carbohydrates-grains, sugars, starches, vegetables, fruits- you are feeding your body a ton of glucose. Your body stores this glucose away as glycogen in the

BONUS:

As a way of saying thank you for purchasing my book, please use your link below to claim your 3 FREE Cookbooks on Health, Fitness & Dieting Instantly

https://bit.ly/2OazEZu

You can also share your link with your friends and families whom you think that can benefit from the cookbooks or you can forward them the link as a gift!

At the end of every bundle can you copy and paste this:

** Remember to use your link to claim your 3 FREE Cookbooks on Health, Fitness & Dieting Instantly

https://bit.ly/2OazEZu

CHAPTER 1

How Ketosis Can Benefit You

If I told you that your body had a natural system for burning fat that you simply weren't utilizing, would you believe me? Most people wouldn't. However, more and more people are coming around to this wonderful diet in what I like to call the low-carb revolution.

The purpose of the ketogenic diet is to retrain your body to run on better fuel. Rather than glucose, your body will learn to run on fat for fuel. Eating this way will place your body in a position wherein it primarily uses fat, rather than sugar for energy.

However, the ketogenic diet is focused on one key concept: *ketosis*. *Ketosis* is, to simply say, an alternative way that the body can burn fuel. When one is in a state of *ketosis*, then they are burning what are called *ketones* for energy, instead of *carbohydrates* like usual. Ketones can be generated from both the body's fat deposits and stores, as well as from ingested fat. This leads us to the first way that ketosis can benefit you: you'll be *less hungry*. We'll talk more about the simple mechanics of weight loss either, but for right now, just understand this: fats burn *slower* than carbs do, which means that you'll be a lot less hungry a lot less often.

Moreover, when you're eating *less* energy than your body is taking out, your body takes energy *directly* from your natural fat stores without any sort of conversion process, meaning that you'll shed pounds like crazy.

When you eat a diet that is heavy in carbohydrates-grains, sugars, starches, vegetables, fruits- you are feeding your body a ton of glucose. Your body stores this glucose away as glycogen in the liver and muscles for later use. The glucose stored in the liver can be used by most systems in the body. The glucose stored in your muscles can only be used by the specific muscle it is stored in. However, your body can store only a limited amount of glucose.

Ketosis can also help with your blood pressure. Ketosis, in a word, causes you to pee – a *lot.* This means that your body requires a lot more water. However, in this heavier urination, you also shed a lot more electrolytes, meaning that your sodium levels can go down massively which will benefit your blood pressure.

The simple idea behind ketosis and the ketogenic diet is simply taking in fat as your main source of cholesterol. One may think that this seems counterintuitive to helping one's blood pressure and general health. However, it's quite the opposite. If you were to run lab tests after having a healthy ketogenic diet for six months, you would find that your lipid levels were higher, your bad cholesterol levels were lower, your good cholesterol levels were higher, and your blood pressure is lower and far more stable than it may have been before. In other words, your blood becomes a lot healthier – and so do you!

CHAPTER 2

What to Expect on Keto

So now that we've talked about what ketosis is, what can you expect on a ketogenic diet? Well, this is actually pretty simple to breakdown.

Firstly, you should expect *rapid weight loss*. People often turn to low-carb diets such as keto because they see the success that others have had with their personal low-carb adventures, and they decide that they'd like to see similar results. This is completely understandable; clinical tests comparing low-carb and low-fat diets have found that people following a low-carb diet will show greater amounts of weight loss at 6 months than those following a low-fat diet.

You will also lose a fair bit of water weight in the first week while your body uses up its glycogen reserves for energy (essentially, what was left over from your body's carbohydrate stores). It's not uncommon for somebody to lose 7 to 10 pounds in their first week in water weight. After this initial period, you should see a steady loss of 1 to 2 pounds per week, potentially more depending upon factors such as age and how your body personally processes energy.

This leads us to the next thing that we have to talk about: *keto flu*. This is an unfortunate affliction that most people starting keto have to deal with. What is essentially happening is a combination of electrolyte imbalance alongside dehydration.

It's simple enough, but can make you feel just like you have the flu! Ketosis, as I said, is diuretic. You're going to have to account for this by drinking a whole lot of water. You're also going to be peeing out a lot of your body's electrolytes, or losing them through other channels in greater amounts. This means that you need to replace them. You'll want to salt your food quite heavily, and also take potassium and magnesium supplements.

If the keto flu gets particularly bad, many find that drinking chicken broth can help them overcome the symptoms of keto flu for a while. This is because chicken broth is rather high in sodium and, of course, is water-based. The combination of these can restore a bit of your body's natural order. In other words, chicken broth can help you to feel better for much the same reason that it did when you drank it as a child to help with the common cold!

One of the reasons that people particularly like low-carb diets for weight loss is because they leave you feeling a lot less hungry. Carbs and fats are burned differently by the body. Fats take longer to process and go further, while carbs tend to be burned very quickly and used in one go. This is why carbs can leave you feeling tired or you get a "sugar high". Fats don't come with that; rather, they leave you feeling full for longer. This means that while other diets might leave you feeling hungry and tired, the ketogenic diet will leave you feeling more energetic and will hardly leave you hungry. It wouldn't be uncommon if you didn't feel like eating breakfast simply because you weren't hungry.

CHAPTER 3

Principles of Weight Loss

I've tried to help a lot of people lose weight, and I've discussed weight loss likewise with a lot of people. I've heard a lot of people make a *lot* of excuses. People could say that, for example, no matter what they do, they just *can't* lose weight for some reason. It's always the same set of excuses - "I simply can't lose weight"; "my body isn't wired for it"; "my metabolism is too slow"; it's the same set of tired diatribes that have little basis in reality.

However, the truth is, weight loss comes down to a simple equation of calories in versus calories out. Although there are certain other factors which may play a part, such as your age or any medications you're on, weight loss, in general, comes down to a simple argument of burned energy. If you eat more calories than you burn, you'll gain weight; if you eat fewer calories than you burn, you'll lose weight.

Your body has a certain amount of calories that it burns as a result of your natural biological processes. This is referred to as your **basal metabolic rate**. This will vary depending on things such as your height, weight, and age. However, these are the calories which you burn without any effort on your end at all!

A lot of people think that you have to be an active person in order to lose weight. This isn't actually the truth. In order to lose weight, you simply have to eat fewer calories than you burn. As long as you eat less than your metabolic rate, you will lose weight. However, it's worth adding that working out is a major boon to your process of getting healthier. Losing weight is only one aspect of a much bigger spider web of increasing your overall physical health. Working out allows you to maintain your muscle mass that you've already got so that your body doesn't burn it off, and also allows you to tone up as you go.

CHAPTER 4

Starting Keto, Step by Step

So now we've talked about the various benefits of starting keto. The question then arises of how to start with keto - and, perhaps more importantly, where to start.

There are two different methods by which you can start keto: you can either start abruptly, or you can ease yourself into it. Many people find that doing the latter is the best means of beating keto flu.

The key thing to remember about starting any diet is that a successful diet isn't a simple dietary change; a successful diet is a holistic lifestyle change. In order to lose weight successfully, you're going to need to change the way you think about food entirely and simply consider it as fuel rather than a leisure activity.

However, combining this alongside a calorie deficit (which most people aren't used to eating at) and an entirely new way of eating can prove to be too much of a shock for many people. This can turn them off of the diet.

If you're not in too much of a rush to lose weight for a wedding or vacation, then consider easing into keto one thing at a time so that you aren't shocking yourself too much.
There are two different forms of keto, known as *strict keto and lazy keto* respectively.

Strict keto is a tightly controlled form of keto which allows you to eat within tightly controlled *macros*. Macros is short for macronutrients - fat, protein, and carbohydrates. The typical diet contains somewhere along the lines of ten percent fat, thirty percent protein, and sixty percent carbohydrates. On strict keto, however, you'd be eating sixty-five percent fat, twenty percent protein, and ten percent carbohydrates.

Lazy keto is simply the maintenance of ketosis by eating less than twenty grams of carbs per day. You can eat at a deficit or not; lazy keto is simply intended for maintenance of the diet and of ketosis.

Which one you decide to do is up to you. Some people work better and are able to stay more on track when they're taking advantage of a tighter regime, such as strict keto. On the other hand, some people find the freedom that lazy keto allows to be better for them personally. Whichever you prefer is the one you should use.

This chapter is specifically dedicated to easing into the ketogenic diet and setting yourself up for success using strict keto.

The first thing that you're going to want to do is figure out what deficit you're wanting to eat at. This can be done quite easily by simply calculating your basal metabolic rate. For calculating your basal metabolic rate, all that you will need are your age, weight, and height. I'm not going to make you do the math, but unfortunately, Amazon isn't kind to links in eBooks - Google "calculate BMR" and you'll be set.

Your basal metabolic rate, as we established in the last chapter, is the number of calories that you burn by simply existing. These are effortless calories. You can lead a sedentary lifestyle and as long as you're eating fewer than this number of calories per day, you *will* lose weight.

At this point, you can also set up a MyFitnessPal account. MyFitnessPal will automatically calculate your basal metabolic rate based on the information you provide. It will also automatically adjust how many calories you should have per day by how many pounds per week you say you'd like to lose. MyFitnessPal lets you log your meals and keep track of how many calories you eat, and you *will* need one if you decide to do strict keto. It's super easy to take anywhere because there's an easy-to-use mobile app for MyFitnessPal on both iOS and Android.

If you opt not to create a MyFitnessPal account and get the application, you're going to need to instead calculate how much of a deficit you need to eat at. I'd recommend only aiming to lose two pounds per week at most. A deficit beyond this is dangerous. There are 3500 calories in one pound, so in order to lose one pound, you must eat at a weekly deficit of 3500 calories or roughly a deficit of 500 calories per day. This means that if your basal metabolic rate is 2200 calories, you'll need to eat only 1700 to 1800 per day in order to lose a pound per week. One and a half pounds per week is a deficit of 750 calories, and two pounds per week is a deficit of 1000 calories. After you account for a 1000 calorie deficit, you're getting into starvation range, which is dangerous.

For the record, should you choose not to follow the steps outlined afterward, you can enter into ketosis by eating below fifty grams of carbs per day. However, the most rapid way is to eat below twenty grams of carbs per day, plus eating sub-twenty allows you to be 100% certain that you're going into ketosis.

Anyhow, moving forward. After figuring out your calorie deficit and learning how to account for the weight that you need to lose, as well as potentially setting up a MyFitnessPal account, you'll be ready to move to the next lesson. The next lesson involves how to read labels specifically for keto. Learning to read calories is not only important but absolutely vital, sure, and you'll want to pay attention to how many calories you consume. However, the best way to ease into keto is by simply becoming *aware* of carbs. Start reading labels of foods that you eat to look for their carbohydrates. This will also get you used to the idea of *net carbs*, which is central to keto. Net carbs are comprised of the carbs you eat which affect blood glucose. This means that the carbohydrates which don't affect blood glucose are unimportant. These may be listed as dietary fiber, sugar alcohols, or any other number of things. If you aren't sure, run a Google search to learn whether or not the term affects blood glucose. To draw the net carbs, you just deduct the grams of dietary fiber and sugar alcohols from the total carbohydrates. The goal on Keto is to eat fewer than twenty grams of net carbs per day; other forms of carbohydrate don't matter, as they don't affect blood sugar, they are simply passed.

The first step to actually transitioning to keto should be to eliminate your sweet tongue. I've found a lot of people from other cultures find it bizarre how many sweets we eat; indeed, once you wean yourself off of sugar, foods that you ate before start to seem *too* sweet by comparison.

You can do this first by eliminating any sodas. Replace them with diet sodas or sparkling water. This is a massive step for a lot of people. Our entire food culture is hugely reliant upon sodas to the point that we have a national coke addiction. Cut it out, and you'll notice a lot of different benefits.

After cutting out sodas, it's time to start cutting down on your snacking habits. Pay attention to them, first and foremost. If you notice that you feel like you're always snacking and subconsciously eating chips all the time, you drastically need to cut down on that. One of the biggest reasons for weight gain is constant snacking and boredom eating.

Again, weight loss has to do with mentality and how you think about food. Most people who are skinny aren't skinny because of their metabolism. Most people who are skinny are so because they don't derive as much pleasure from food, and see it more as fuel. You need to start thinking about food as fuel if you want to see a reasonable change in your weight.

There's no reason to boredom eat, whatsoever. Eating should be a conscious and mindful activity. Think about what you're eating, when you are. Eat slowly and consider the taste and feeling. You will feel fuller.

I'm sorry, but there's no compromise on this one. You either quit constantly snacking, or you aren't going to lose weight. It's a bad habit and one that should be broken. It's one thing if instead of three meals per day, you snack throughout the day, but if that's not the case then you need to cut out snacks. Calories add up too quickly. The only case in which you can make an exception is if you lead an active lifestyle.

After cutting out snacking, you're even closer to losing weight using keto. The next thing you're going to want to cut out is all dairy aside from heavy cream, half and half, and cheese without sugar added. This means that if you're a big milk drinker, you're going to be cutting it out at this point - sorry! It also means that if you eat cereal for breakfast on a daily basis you're going to need to find an alternative, such as eggs and bacon.

Next, you're going to want to cut out bread and other grains. This means you'll be saying goodbye to bread, rice, oatmeal, and any related foods. This can be a hard step, just consider breaking your portions in half at first. Order burgers with one bun instead of two, for example.

After cutting out bread and grains, you're most of the way there. The last big thing to cut out is fruit. While there are some fruits, like blueberries, which have a relatively low carb count, it may be easier to cut them out entirely. They serve as too much of a temptation and it becomes very difficult to constantly measure out exact servings.

At this point, you've dwindled it down to meat, cheese, vegetables, and nuts. Good. You're now, mostly, eating keto. One more thing you'll want to be wary of is that you should primarily be eating leafy vegetables and greens. Beware of lentils and beans as they have a huge number of carbs. Additionally, this is when you need to start cutting starches out of your diet almost entirely. Starches are things like potatoes. You do not need them, and they only serve to give you unnecessary carbs. Don't worry though; almost every starch has a nice keto replacement.

Transitioning to keto can be rather difficult; this isn't supposed to be a process that you undertake all at once. It can be nauseating if you try to do so. Rather, take a week on each step so you slowly adjust. Again, this is a *lifestyle* change, not just a diet.

CHAPTER 5

Sample Keto Recipes

Here are sample recipes you can use when you're starting off with keto.

Southwest Bacon Omelet

You'll need:

- 3 eggs
- 4 strips bacon
- ½ small onion
- 1 jalapeño
- ¼ cup cheddar cheese, shredded

1. Grill bacon in a skillet until cooked. Remove from the skillet and let it cool.

2. Chop jalapeño and onion, then sauté in bacon grease. Remove from the heat and place with the bacon.

3. Add olive oil to the pan in order to coat, then drain off the fat combination.

4. Crack and scramble eggs then place in a pan. Allow to cook for a moment, then add all ingredients.

5. Fold over omelet and let it cook for 1 minute on either side.

6. Serve and enjoy!

Calories: 630

Fat: 60g

Protein: 22g

Carbs: 4g

Zucchini Circles with Olive Garlic Sauce

You'll need:

- 2 zucchinis
- 2 oz smoked cheddar cheese
- ½ large onion
- 1 clove garlic
- 1 jalapeño
- Fresh cilantro
- ½ tomato
- Olive oil

1. Cut zucchini into thin circles. Roast 1 zucchini in the oven at 350 degrees for 30 minutes, flipping halfway. Set other to the side.

2. Meanwhile, prepare onion, garlic, and jalapeño by chopping.

3. Grill onion, garlic, and jalapeño in olive oil.

4. Add in roasted zucchini and grill together.

5. Add salt and pepper liberally.

6. Add smoked cheddar cheese and olive oil. Let cheddar melt. Squeeze tomato to get juices out. Set aside and chop remaining flesh.

7. Remove from the heat. Add cilantro, remaining zucchini, and tomato. Stir.

Calories: 470

Fat: 45g

Protein: 15g

Carbs: 6g

Crispy Flaxseed Waffles

You'll need:

- 2 cups ground flaxseed
- 1 tablespoon baking powder
- 1 teaspoon sea salt
- 5 tablespoons finely ground flaxseed with 15 tablespoons of warm water. Let it sit for 5 minutes until it's gooey (to replace eggs).
- ½ cup water
- ⅓ cup avocado oil or extra-virgin olive oil or melted coconut oil
- 2 teaspoons ground cinnamon

1. Heat waffle maker to medium high

2. In a large bowl, combine flax seed with baking powder and sea salt. Whisk to combine fully and set aside.

3. Add egg substitute, water and oil to a blender and blend on high for 30 seconds, until foamy.

4. Transfer liquid mixture to the bowl with the flaxseed mixture.

5. Stir to incorporate. The mixture will be very fluffy. Once incorporated, allow to sit for 3 minutes.

6. Toss in ground cinnamon.

7. Divide mixture into 4 servings. Scoop each; one at a time, onto the preheated waffle maker and close the top. Cook till done and repeat with remaining batter.

8. Serve warm or freeze in an air-tight container for a couple of weeks.

Calories: 297 Fat: 16g Protein: 8.9g Carbs: 8.4g

Those are just sample recipes to help get you started. Get creative in the kitchen!

CHAPTER 6

Sample Keto Shopping List

There are a lot of different keto recipes out there, so it's very difficult to pin down a shopping list or an exact set of items that you'll need. However, there are a few sample guidelines you should absolutely follow. The first is that you're going to want primarily products which, obviously, are low carb and high fat. This will include meats, cheeses, and nuts. However, you're also going to want to grab a lot of leafy greens and vegetables that you can cook up and prepare.

Here is a sample list that you can use when doing ketogenic shopping:

- Lunch meat
- Ground beef
- Bacon
- Raw chicken, pork
- Cheddar cheese
- Mozzarella cheese
- Cream cheese
- Colby jack cheese
- Butter (grass-fed preferably)
- Olive oil
- Heavy cream -Half and half
- Coffee or tea
- Lots of water
- Spinach
- Broccoli
- Cauliflower
- Jalapeño pepper
- Yellow onion (use sparingly)

- Tomato (use sparingly)
- Garlic
- Eggs

Of course, you may also find recipes online that you'd like to try making. These will add items to your necessary grocery shopping. These are just basic requirements that will push you happy and healthy through your first week or two of keto.

CHAPTER 7

What to Eat and What Not to Eat

One of the hardest things about keto can be learning what you can and cannot eat. Indeed, this can be a little bit difficult. However, it's not totally horrible. It just takes a little bit of effort!

First, as should be perfectly clear, you aren't going to be eating any fruits or sugars. If something contains either, you aren't going to eat it. The same goes for starches. Don't eat any potatoes, sweet potatoes, or plant roots in general. These are loaded with carbs and will make your blood sugar skyrocket. I've got no doubt that part of the reason America has such a health crisis right now is our obsession with starches!

I'm sure by now you've figured out that your keto diet will consist primarily of meat, cheese, nuts, and any products coming thereof. However, there's a bit of a devil in the details here. First off, be sure that you're eating more than a fair amount of leafy greens. These are your primary source of vitamins and important nutrients, and make a great vehicle for a variance. Meat and cheese can get repetitive. Vegetables, however, can be prepared in any number of different ways!

Also, it can be tempting to cut corners and eat ketogenically solely on beef franks and Vienna sausage. However, avoid processed foods. They are absolutely loaded to the brim with sodium and all sorts of other disgusting things which can make your blood sugar skyrocket. By eating fresh meats and cheeses, you can ensure that you aren't ingesting way too much sodium. You're also making your time on Keto far more enjoyable- we all know fresher food tastes better, and on keto, it costs about the same. So embrace it! Eat fresh deli meats whenever possible.

One last thing: fried food is generally not okay because it's almost always fried in breadcrumbs or a wheat-based batter. This, obviously, can add unnecessary carbs to your diet.

Some people, when they do keto, try to mimic their current eating style by finding replacement foods for their usual foods. This may or may not be the thing you want to do. It's possible, for example, that by making a delicious keto pizza, you get cravings for real pizza, and likewise for any keto sweet replacements. However, there's also the possibility that these can make your transition easier. I'm not going to label these as a do eat or do not eat. It depends on your personal fortitude and, much like strict keto versus lazy keto, what you're trying to do for yourself. If you want keto to be a holistic lifestyle change for the long-term, it may be worth looking. If you just want to hit a goal weight, it may be best to avoid these, as it will take your eyes off of the prize.

Those are basic rules for eating even on while keto. They can keep you happy and healthy as you try to chug your way through your weight loss.

CHAPTER 8

Tips for Eating Out on Keto

One of the hardest things about starting a new diet can be learning to eat in public while you're on it. This process can be painstaking but it doesn't have to be. There are some things that you'll kind of grow into as you learn how keto works and figure out intuitively what you're going to be able to eat - and likewise, what you won't be able to eat.

However, here are some general tips for different cuisines that I've discovered.

American food is a breeze, fortunately. If you go to a steakhouse, you can order any given meat on the menu. Steamed broccoli is always a safe side, and you can salt or butter it to your content. If they don't have any other keto friendly sides, just double up on steamed broccoli.

Diners are easy as well. Often, diners are willing to replace hash browns and other foods that aren't particularly keto friendly with a different side. The classic breakfast of eggs and bacon or sausage is a great go-to, and nothing beats a good steak and eggs.

Coffeehouses are increasingly becoming prevalent as a part of the daily grind. Unfortunately, dropping everything that you know and love - like your caramel macchiato - can be a massive pain. However, you don't have to give it up entirely, fortunately! You can easily get a coffee with cream and sugar-free vanilla syrup. If you want your espresso fix, then espresso is perfectly keto. You can get a Caffè Americano with cream and sugar-free vanilla and it will taste a fair bit like the milky coffee drinks you know and love while clocking in at very few calories.

Mexican food can be harder to eat on Keto. It can be really tempting to eat chips and salsa but you need to resist that temptation and tough through the meal! Your waistline will thank you later. One thing you can always get at a Mexican restaurant is a taco salad. Simply ask that they hold the shell and you'll be all set.

Vietnamese food can be really hard to eat on Keto. Your best option if you're going out to eat Vietnamese is simply to get pho without any noodles.

Japanese food is absolutely delicious, centered around freshness and delicate flavors. However, eating Japanese food while maintaining your keto status can be a difficult task in and of itself. The best option is almost always going to be sashimi. Sashimi is simply super fresh raw fish, and super delicious, too. You'll hardly have something better in your life, so it's well worth ordering in lieu of sushi.

Chinese food is almost impossible to eat out on, unfortunately. Avoid going to Chinese restaurants as much as you can. If you must, then avoid anything with a sauce as the sauces often contain cornstarch. Cornstarch is loaded with carbs. They also frequently contain sugar.

Italian food is likewise ridiculously hard - the core of Italian dining lies in pasta and bread products. Needless to say, it's almost impossible to find keto food to eat when you're at an Italian restaurant. If you're forced to eat at an Italian restaurant, do what you can to find something based around meat and cheese with minimal sugars and starches.

It's impossible to cover every cuisine, but these are the ones I have the most experience with. I hope that these tips aid you with eating out!

Conclusion

Thank for making it through to the end of this book, let's hope it was informative and able to provide you with all of the tools you need to achieve your goals whatever they may be. The next step is to take all of this and apply it to your personal life. Conquer keto and conquer your figure! Finally, if you found this book useful in any way, a review on Amazon is always appreciated!

The Complete Mediterranean Diet For Beginners

CHAPTER 1

THE CHARACTERISTICS OF THE MEDITERRANEAN DIET

The Mediterranean diet doesn't incorporate anything fancy or complicated into its eating habits, instead focusing on the basics of eating healthy with a dash of olive oil and a glass or two of red wine added in for flavor. Broadly speaking it features as its chief components the traditional foods of the countries surrounding the Mediterranean Sea.

The diet includes plenty of healthy whole grains, fish, vegetables and fruits, while limiting unhealthy fats and processed foods. While these can all be said to be part of many healthy diets, there are variations in the Mediterranean Diet that can especially make a difference to those who are dealing with an increased risk of heart disease.

Crucial components

In general, the Mediterranean Diet emphasizes the regular consumption of plant-based foods including nuts, legumes, whole grains, vegetables and fruits. It also recommends switching out butter for other types of healthy fats such as canola or olive oil. Likewise, it recommends making a habit or replacing herbs and spices for flavoring foods rather than salt. As a rule, you should only eat red meat a few times each month, while also eating fish and poultry each at least twice per week.

When it comes to grains, nuts, vegetables and fruits, the number of servings you should aim for in a given day should reach Grecian levels. Greeks tend to eat only small amounts of red meat while consuming as many as nine servings of vegetables and fruits each day. Grains in this region tend to be of the whole grain variety and rarely contain any trans fats. The biggest difference with that region's dietary habits and the standard Western Diet is that they use olive oil for dipping bread in rather than margarine or butter, both of which contain saturated and trans fats. Another Mediterranean Diet alternative to butter for dipping is tahini sauce.

In general, you are going to want to strive for between seven and ten servings of fruits and vegetables per day. You are going to want to aim for high-quality whole grain bread and cereal and work more pasta and whole grain rice into your diet. These foods are rich in antioxidants and can benefit your body in a wide variety of different ways.

Nuts are another common part of the Mediterranean Diet. Nuts are comprised of about 80 percent healthy fats which makes them a great post-workout snack. They are extremely high in calories, however, so a little is going to go a long way. In generally, you are going to want to stick to a handful or two each day, and avoid anything that is heavily salted or honey-roasted.

When it comes to dealing with fat, the Mediterranean Diet doesn't focus on limiting total fat consumption and instead focuses on substituting good fats for bad fats. As such, the Mediterranean Diet discourages the consumption of hydrogenated oils which contain trans fats along with saturated fats, both of which are known to actively contribute to heart disease.

The Mediterranean Diet is also known for its heavy use of olive oil as its primary fat source. Olive oil provides monosaturated fat, which is a type of fat that is known to reduce bad cholesterol levels when it is used in place of more traditional trans or saturated fats. Virgin and extra virgin olive oils are often recommended as they are the least processed forms of the substance which means that they contain more of the beneficial plant compounds that generate the antioxidant effects that make the Mediterranean Diet so effective.

Additionally, polyunsaturated fats and monounsaturated fats, like those found in nuts and canola oil, contains a beneficial version of the omega-3 fatty acid known as linolenic acid. This fatty acid is known to lower triglycerides and decrease blood clotting and is generally associated with a decrease risk for heart attack. Likewise, fatty fish including salmon, tuna, albacore, sardines, herring, lake trout and mackerel are all known to be great sources of omega-3 fatty acids and the heavy consumption of fish is believed to be one of the things that makes the diet so effective overall. It should go without saying that you are going to want to cook the fish in the healthiest manner possible, no frying allowed.

Finally, while wine isn't considered a mandatory part of the diet, regular, and moderate, consumption of alcohol is known to be beneficial for a number of reasons. The average Mediterranean Diet tends to include about five ounces of wine per day for women and 10 ounces for men under the age of 65. If you have a family or personal history with alcohol abuse or liver or heart disease then it is strongly encouraged that you leave wine off of the menu.

CHAPTER 2

WHY CHOOSE THE MEDITERRANEAN DIET

Low in sugar and processed foods: As the diet is primarily made up of ingredients that are as close to nature as possible, this means that the foods you are going to be eating on the Mediterranean Diet will naturally be low in sugar, GMOs and other unnatural ingredients that are known to cause so much havoc within the human body when they are consumed on a regular basis.

Beyond plant-based foods, the Mediterranean Diet promotes the consumption of only a small amount of heavier meals and meats in general, instead favoring lighter and healthier options. This then naturally leads to weight loss and helps to improve omega-3 fatty acid intake, heart health and cholesterol.

Promotes healthy weight loss: When it comes to losing weight without feeling hungry, the Mediterranean Diet is a great way to go about doing so. The diet has the benefit of being both healthy and sustainable in the long-term meaning it is not so much a temporary fix, but a permanent lifestyle change. The focus on high quality proteins means that the diet can help keep you feeling full for longer, despite consuming fewer calories overall while also including additional benefits in the form of omega-3s and probiotics.

Furthermore, dairy, fish and red meat that is grass-fed contain high amounts of other types of healthy fatty acids that the body needs to help you feel full, control blood sugar, increase your overall energy level, improve your mood and moderate weight gain. If you are looking for a vegetarian or vegan option the diet still provides lots of protein options in the forms of whole grains and legumes.

Heart healthy choices: Studies show that sticking to the Mediterranean Diet, especially omega-3 rich foods and those high in monosaturated fats, is known to decrease mortality rate significantly, especially when it comes to issues related to heart disease. This is due to the linolenic acid found in olive oil which has been linked to decreasing the risk of cardiac death by as much as 30 percent and the risk of sudden death due to a cardiac event by as much as 45 percent.

What's more, research also shows that if the blood pressure of those who consume sunflower oil is compared to that of those who are consuming primarily extra-virgin olive oil, those who regularly consume the olive oil are going to have significantly lower results. It is also known to be beneficial when it comes to decreasing the effects of hypertension as it causes the body to generate more nitric acid which serves to counteract the process. Likewise, it also promotes oxidation while improving endothelial function which serves to counteract the condition.

Cancer fighting: The Mediterranean Diet is known to help combat the growth of a variety of cancer cells due to the way in which it provides the body with a measured amount of omega-3 and omega-6 fatty acids along with high amounts of polyphenols, antioxidants and fiber. As plant-based foods are a cornerstone of the Mediterranean

Diet, then it can be said that eating in this way protects the very DNA from damage by decreasing the chances of cell mutation and inflammation which, in turn, helps to decrease the growth of tumors.

There are also studies that show that olive oil could very well prove to be a natural cure for bowel and colon cancer. It has been shown to decrease the development of cancer cells in these regions as it lowers inflammation while also decreasing the rate of oxidative stress the body is under.

Helps get diabetes under control: The Mediterranean Diet is known to provide relief for diseases that are based around chronic inflammation such as type 2 diabetes and metabolic syndrome. One of the reasons that this is the case is the fact that the diet helps to control the excess production of insulin that is common in these issues. By regulating blood sugar levels through a balance of whole foods containing carbohydrates that are low in sugar, quality proteins and healthy fatty acids, the diet allows the body to burn fat more efficiently while maintaining more energy in the process.

Enhances cognitive processes: Recent research suggests that the Mediterranean Diet may prove to be a natural cure for Alzheimer's disease as well as dementia. These types of cognitive disorders are known to occur when the brain isn't receiving enough dopamine.

Luckily, healthy fats such as that found in nuts and olive oil, when combined with the anti-inflammatory power of fruits and vegetables are known to fight off this type of cognitive decline. This occurs because the diet helps to counter the effectives that free radicals, toxicity and inflammation can have on the brain after a prolonged period of time.

CHAPTER 3

A BRIEF HISTORY OF THE MEDITERRANEAN DIET

The first version of the Mediterranean Diet was theorized in the 1970s by Ancel Keys, a biologist from America and his wife Margaret Keys a chemist and his writer and collaborator. However, it failed to gain widespread acceptance until it was reintroduced in 1993 by the European Office of the World Health Organization and the Harvard School of Public Health at a conference in Cambridge Massachusetts. Based on the dietary traditions of Greece, Crete and Southern Italy from around 1960, the original study found that rates in this area when it came to chronic diseases were some of the lowest in the entire world. Likewise, the life expectancy of the average adult in this area was among the longest in the world, despite the fact that many of the people in the region didn't have access to reliable healthcare.

The key to this longevity, the scientists who introduced it argued, was that the diet had resisted what at the time was approximately 50 years of efforts to modernize food that had been taking place at the time in many industrialized countries. These trends in modernization tended to lead towards a diet that contained more beef and other animal products, while at the same time overall fewer fruits and vegetables and a much higher concentration of processed foods.

On the contrary, the diet of the region in question continued to consist mainly of vegetables, fruits, whole grains and fish, along with plenty of olive oil and wine, of course. Other vital elements of the Mediterranean Diet, the study insisted included plenty of daily exercise along with the practice of eating meals in groups and taking the time to more fully appreciate food before consuming it. This, in turn, naturally leads to a more leisurely meal pace which means that food has more time to pass through the body before the meal is complete, leading to smaller portion sizes as well.

While it may seem odd today, with millionaires paying untold sums for third world delicacies and celebrities subsisting on water, cayenne pepper and lemon juice, one of the biggest reasons that the Mediterranean Diet failed to catch on initially was that it was seen as a diet for the poor. In fact, when Keys did the initial study, Portugal was also listed as one of the main regional contributors to the diet. However, the leader of Portugal didn't want his country to be listed among the countries polled for this diet of the poor so the country was stricken from the dietary record.

Soon after it began to gain popularity in the mainstream, a number of companies from the agriculture and food sectors in Barcelona got together to essentially promote their brand while telling the people that abandoning the traditional eating habits of their people would do them little good in the long run. This group became the Association for the Advancement of the Mediterranean Diet in late 1995 with the stated mission of encouraging the consumption of traditional Mediterranean products for the health benefits of all.

This group then joined with a number of other similarly themed organizations to form the Mediterranean Diet Foundation in 1996. The mission of the foundation is to promote keen insight into the benefits surrounding the Mediterranean Diet when it comes to gastronomical, cultural, historical and health aspects. Furthermore, the foundation aims to disseminate scientific findings regarding the diet and the ways it can benefit the health of people around the world.

Since its inception, the FDM has been involved in a wide variety of activities, starting with the spreading of a wide variety of research through the use of biennial conferences that take place during large international food exhibitions. At the Alimentaria conference in 1996, the Barcelona Declaration on the Mediterranean Diet was signed by the FDM, the Barcelona City Countil, Fish and Food, the Spanish Ministry of Agriculture and the Food and Agriculture Organization. Later that same year the Grande Covian award was created to recognize professionals who had contributed greatly to the study of the Mediterranean Diet.

The FDM has also been granting honorary diplomas since the start of the 00s to individuals who have proven that they excel when it comes to their contributions in the social and cultural sphere when it comes to promoting the Mediterranean Diet and Mediterranean culture. Individuals recognized in this way so far include Juan Antonio Corbalán, Bigas Luna, Joan Manuel Serrat, Georges Moustaki and the great Ferran Adrià. These awards are given out during each biennial conference at the same time as the Grande Covian. The group has also formed a partnership with the FOOD Program which is working to influence dietary changes in the workplace and is specifically targeting habits and lifestyles that are directly known to lead to obesity.

CHAPTER 4

THE MEDITERRANEAN DIET PYRAMID

The Mediterranean Diet Pyramid was developed and released at the same time as the Mediterranean Diet was being reintroduced to the public in the 1990s. It sums up the way that the diet suggests that followers break up their eating patterns, making it easier to determine the types of foods you should eat each day. The pyramid is, unsurprisingly, also closely tied to areas of olive oil cultivation in the Mediterranean. The Mediterranean Diet Pyramid is broken into monthly, weekly and daily units, but does not list serving sizes other than to note to keep meals reasonably sized.

The original Mediterranean Diet Pyramid was created using then current nutritional research as a means of representing a well-rounded Mediterranean diet. It recommended potatoes, grains, bulgur, polenta, couscous, rice, pasta and breads with every meal. Fruits, vegetables and olive oil were recommended on a daily basis along with smaller amounts of yogurt and cheese. It recommended fish and poultry a few times a week and sweets and red meat sparingly, only a few times a month. Red wine was also recommended in moderation. A new layer added to the bottom of the pyramid to account for the need for daily exercise was also added in 2000 as fears about a nationwide obesity epidemic first started materializing. While the original graph was nothing but simple words, the pyramid was soon updated with various graphics to ensure that the foods at each level were clear.

While the graphics were updated over the years, the science underlying the Mediterranean Diet Pyramid remained the same for the next fifteen years. For that year's Mediterranean Diet Conference, however, Harvard scientists decided to review the pyramid in light of nutritional findings that had come to light in the previous decade and a half of academic research. One of the biggest changes to the pyramid at this time was the addition of spices and herbs as a replacement for salt when it comes to maximizing taste. It also serves to make the pyramid more accurate as these spices and herbs contribute significantly to the national identities of many of the dishes that are a core of the Mediterranean Diet.

Additionally, the scientists changed the placement of fish on the pyramid and also added shellfish to the list, noting that the increase to at least twice a week would better serve to emphasize the benefits that are gained when omega-6 fatty acids and omega-3 fatty acids are in balance with one another. An advisory board was also convened which came to a consensus on several other aspects of the Mediterranean Diet Pyramid as well. These changes primarily centered around gathering olive oil, olives, seeds, legumes, nuts, grains, vegetables into a single group to make it clear that they are all on the same page when it comes to health benefits. The goal with this change was to also draw extra attention to the key role that these foods should play in the health-promoting pattern of the diet and also to put all of these items onto equal footing.

This update to the terms of the pyramid prompted a visual update in 2009 with the help of artist George Middleton. He created an entirely new graphic to represent the pyramid that reflects the current most effective grouping of foods according to the experts. The pyramid now shows physical activity, eating with others and enjoying your meals at the bottom, followed by a very large space for fruits, vegetables, whole grains, olive oil, nuts, beans, legumes, seeds, spice and herbs to be consumed with every meal. Above that is fish and other seafood which should be consumed at least twice each week. Next is yogurt, cheese, eggs and poultry which can be consumed multiple times in a week. At the top is still sweets and red meat which should be consumed just a few times each month. Finally, it recommends drinking lots of water and wine in moderation.

CHAPTER 5

TIPS TO SUPERCHARGE WEIGHT LOSS

Never skip a meal: While it may seem to make sense that skipping the occasional meal should promote weight loss, after all you are eating fewer calories in a given day, the fact is the opposite is true. This is because your body gets into a habit of taking in and burning calories throughout the day based on your average eating patterns and missing a meal gums up the works. Rather than taking in and burning calories as anticipated, your body now needs to stretch what was already available further than it was planning to which means it will have to play catchup later on. This, in turn, means that skipping that meal will likely cause you to hold onto more weight that day, not less as your body will try and hold onto everything it can until it knows just what is going on.

You should always start your day off with a healthy and nutritious breakfast as this will kick your metabolism into gear at the start of the day, keeping it in the habit of not holding onto any additional fat throughout the day. Ideally you will want to split your day up into three moderate meals and then three light snacks so that you are eating about every three hours. This will ensure that once your metabolism gets going in the morning, it won't stop, burning more calories overall throughout the day than you would otherwise. It is important to watch what you consume with this strategy, however, as choosing unhealthy snacks will negate any work that you are doing by sticking to the Mediterranean Diet.

Lift weights: Your body will naturally burn more fat if it is full of muscle instead of just more fat. As such, the more muscle you build on the regular, the more calories your body will burn every day, even while at rest.

Muscle burns fat which means that your metabolism will also increase if your overall muscle mass is higher. This means that if you start weight training then you will likely see the fat melt off faster than you might think as you are now burning fat while exercising, and then burning more fat than ever before, even while at rest. In order to take things up to the next level, you will also want to add in a mixture of high intensity workouts to your regular exercise routine. These high intensity workouts are usually 30 minutes or less and include a quick burst of cardio in addition to the weights. Adding it in at random intervals will make it hard for your body to anticipate the extra effort required which will cause your metabolism to go into overdrive as a result. It is important to not overdo it, however, as high intensity workouts can easily lead to strain.

Drink the right caffeinated beverages: When consumed without any additives, both coffee and tea can help you jump-start your metabolism. The one thing you should never drink, however, is soda, even if it doesn't have any calories. The wide variety of artificial ingredients in diet sodas can have a wide variety of unpredictable effects on the body, including causing you to hold onto fat that you otherwise would have already ditched. Rather than stick with artificial stuff, you should focus on herbal teas such as Skinny Teatox which can really help you knock off the extra pounds. This is the case because the herbs in these teas are known to improve the rate at which your body metabolizes food while also decreasing the response that fat cells have to sugar. Finally, they are also known to improve the way that fat cells react to insulin which, in turn, helps to aid in digestion and increase the overall functionality of the metabolism.

When it comes to coffee, you should drink it black as the antioxidant catechins it contains have been proven to add a boost to the metabolic system. What's more, if you drink a double shot of espresso before you exercise you are likely to burn as many as

20 percent more calories than you would otherwise. You will see some benefit if you drink your cup of Joe directly after exercising as well, though the effects will be lessened.

Embrace the cold: The more energy that your body requires in order to normalize its temperature, the higher your metabolism will remain overall. Essentially, what this means is that if you exercise in the cold your body will be required to burn more energy just to reach its core required temperature. The colder it is when you exercise the greater the amount of bad fat that you will burn in the interim. You can also increase your metabolism in this fashion by drinking lots of ice water and regularly taking ice-cold showers.

Drink more water: Water is a crucial element of life and, like most aspects of the way the body functions, the metabolism cannot work properly without enough water. The average person is more dehydrated than they should be more than 70 percent of the time. Don't think you are in that majority? Ask yourself if you are thirsty right now. If the answer is yes then you are already dehydrated. Ideally you are going to want to aim to drink a gallon of water each day. This is a gallon of water a day, pure, water with additives doesn't count. The more you can manage in a day, the more smoothly your metabolism will run at all times and the more weight you will lose every day.

Eat more spicy foods: The capsaicin spice, what causes the heat in most spicy foods is also known to increase your metabolism. This is due to the fact that eating it causes the body's internal temperature to increase which means that it needs to work harder to remain parity with the outside temperature. As a general rule, if a meal is hot enough to make you start to sweat, then it is going to be hot enough to increase your metabolism as well.

CHAPTER 6

10 TOP MEDITERRANEAN RECIPES

1: Grecian Chicken Pasta

This recipe needs 15 minutes to prepare, 15 minutes to cook and will make 6 servings.

- Protein: 32.6 grams
- Carbs: 70 grams
- Fats: 11.4 grams
- Calories: 488

What to Use
- Olive oil (1 T)
- Red onion (.5 c chopped)
- Linguine (16 oz.)
- Pepper (as desired)
- Salt (as desired)
- Lemons (2 wedged)
- Oregano (2 tsp. dried)
- Lemon juice (2 T)
- Parsley (3 T chopped)
- Feta cheese (.5 c crumbled)
- Tomato (1 chopped)
- Marinated artichoke hearts (14 oz. chopped, drained)
- Chicken breast (1 lb. cubed)
- Garlic (2 cloves crushed)

What to Do

• Fill a large pot with water and a pinch of salt before placing it on the stove on top of a burner that has been turned to a high heat. Once the water boils, add in the pasta and let it cook until it is still firm but just starting to become tender, which should take approximately 8 minutes.

- Add the olive oil to a skillet before placing it on top of a burner turned to a high/medium heat. Place the garlic and onion into the skillet and let it cook for approximately 2 minutes until it begins to be fragrant.
- Mix in the chicken and stir regularly until the chicken ceases to be pink and all of its juices are clear, this should take approximately 5 minutes. The chicken should end up with an internal temperature of 165F.
- Turn the burner to a low/medium heat before adding in the pasta, oregano, lemon juice, parsley, feta cheese, tomato and artichoke hearts. Let the results cook while stirring for roughly 2 minutes.
- Remove the skillet from the burner, season as desired and garnish using the lemon prior to serving.

2: Feta and Spinach Bake

This recipe needs 10 minutes to prepare, 12 minutes to cook and will make 6 servings.

- Protein: 11.6 grams
- Carbs: 41.6 grams
- Fats: 17.1 grams
- Calories: 350

What to Use
- Pepper (as desired)
- Salt (as desired)
- Extra virgin olive oil (2 T)
- Parmesan cheese (2 T)
- Feta cheese (.5 c crumbled)
- Mushrooms (4 sliced)
- Spinach (1 bunch chopped, rinsed)
- Roma tomatoes (2 chopped)
- Whole wheat pita (6, 6 in.)
- Sun-dried tomato peso (6 oz.)

What to Do
- Ensure your oven is heated to 350F.
- Top one side of each pita using the sun-dried tomato peso before placing them face-up on a baking sheet. Top with mushrooms, spinach and tomatoes before adding the parmesan and feta cheese and topping with olive oil and seasoning as desired.
- Place the baking sheet in the oven and let the pita bake until they are crisp which should take approximately 10 minutes.
- Quarter the pita prior to serving.

3: White Beans, Tomatoes and Greek Pasta

This recipe needs 10 minutes to prepare, 15 minutes to cook and will make 4 servings.

- Protein: 23.4 grams
- Carbs: 79 grams
- Fats: 5.9 grams
- Calories: 460

What to Use
- Pepper (as desired)
- Salt (as desired)
- Feta cheese (.5 c crumbled)
- Penne pasta (8 oz.)
- Spinach (10 oz. chopped, washed)
- Cannellini beans (19 oz. rinsed, drained)
- Italian style tomatoes (14.5 oz. diced)

What to Do
- Fill a large pot with water and a pinch of salt before placing it on the stove on top of a burner that has been turned to a high heat. Once the water boils, add in the pasta and let it cook until it is just starting to become tender which should take about 8 minutes.
- While the pasta is cooking, add the olive oil to a skillet before placing it on top of a burner turned to a high/medium heat. Add in the beans and the tomatoes and let everything boil. After this

occurs, reduce the heat to low/medium and let everything simmer for 10 minutes.
• Add in the spinach and let it cook for 2 minutes or until it starts to wilt, stirring regularly.
• Plate pasta and top with sauce and crumbled feta prior to serving.

4: Cannellini Beans and Pasta

This recipe needs 5 minutes to prepare, 20 minutes to cook and will make 8 servings.

- Protein: 8.2 grams
- Carbs: 30.5 grams
- Fats: 4.2 grams
- Calories: 185

What to Use
- Pepper (as desired)
- Salt (as desired)
- Seashell pasta (.25 lbs.)
- Basil (1 tsp.)
- Parsley (.25 c)
- Cannellini beans (15 oz.)
- Low-sodium chicken broth (3 c)
- Tomatoes (14.5 oz. stewed)
- Garlic (3 cloves minced)
- Onion (1 c chopped)
- Extra virgin olive oil (2 T)

What to Do
• Add the oil to a Dutch oven that is at least 4 quarts before placing it on top of a medium heat. After it warms, add in the garlic and onions and let them cook for approximately 5 minutes or until the onion is nice and tender.
• Mix in the basil, parsley, chicken broth, tomatoes and cannellini beans and season as desired before turning the heat to high and

letting everything boil. Let everything boil for 60 seconds and then turn the heat to low/medium and let everything simmer for 10 minutes with the Dutch oven covered.

• Mix in the pasta and let everything simmer for about 10 minutes until the pasta is extremely tender.

5: Sicilian Spaghetti

This recipe needs 10 minutes to prepare, 5 minutes to cook and will make 8 servings.

- Protein: 12.4 grams
- Carbs: 53.6 grams
- Fats: 9.8 grams
- Calories: 355

What to Use
- Pepper (as desired)
- Salt (as desired)
- Extra virgin olive oil (2 T)
- Parmesan cheese (4 T grated)
- Parsley (1 c)
- Bread crumbs (1 c)
- Anchovy filets (2 oz. chopped)
- Garlic (3 cloves crushed)
- Olive oil (4 T)
- Spaghetti (1 lb.)

What to Do
• Fill a large pot with water and a pinch of salt before placing it on the stove on top of a burner that has been turned to a high heat. Once the water boils, add in the pasta and let it cook for approximately 8 minutes and has reach an al dente state. Drain the pasta and set aside.

• While the pasta cooks, add the olive oil to a skillet before placing it on top of a burner turned to a high/medium heat. Place the

garlic and anchovies into the skillet and let them cook for approximately 2 minutes, stirring constantly.
- Add in the breadcrumbs before turning the heat off on the burner. Add in the parsley and season as desired before mixing well.
- Toss the pasta and the sauce together and top with cheese prior to serving.

6: Broccoli and Cavatelli

This recipe needs 10 minutes to prepare, 20 minutes to cook and will make 12 servings.

- Protein: 10.2 grams
- Carbs: 47.6 grams
- Fats: 10.3 grams
- Calories: 317

What to Use
- Pepper (as desired)
- Salt (as desired)
- Extra virgin olive oil (.5 c)
- Parmesan cheese (2 T)
- Red pepper flakes (1 tsp.)
- Cavatelli pasta (1.5 lbs.)
- Garlic (3 cloves minced)
- Broccoli (3 heads florets)

What to Do
- Fill a large pot with water before adding in the broccoli and placing it on top of the stove over a burner turned to a high heat. Let the broccoli blanch for roughly 5 minutes before draining the broccoli and setting aside
- Refill the large pot with water and a pinch of salt before placing it on the stove on top of a burner that has been turned to a high heat. Once the water boils, add in the pasta and let it cook for approximately 8 minutes until it has reached an al dente state.

Once it has finished cooking, drain it and add it to a large serving bowl.
- While the pasta is cooking, add the olive oil to a skillet before placing it on top of a burner turned to a high/medium heat. Place the garlic into the skillet and let it sauté until it starts to turn a golden hue, take care to ensure it doesn't burn. Mix in the broccoli and let it cook for about 10 minutes, stirring occasionally, the broccoli should be slightly tender but still largely crisp.
- Toss the broccoli with the pasta and season well. Top with parmesan cheese prior to serving.

7: Shrimp and Penne

This recipe needs 10 minutes to prepare, 20 minutes to cook and will make 8 servings.

- Protein: 24.5 grams
- Carbs: 48.5 grams
- Fats: 8.5 grams
- Calories: 385

What to Use
- Pepper (as desired)
- Salt (as desired)
- Extra virgin olive oil (2 T)
- Parmesan cheese (1 c grated)
- Shrimp (1 lb. deveined, peeled)
- Tomatoes (29 oz. diced)
- White wine (.25 c)
- Garlic (1 T chopped)
- Red onion (.25 c)
- Olive oil (2 T)
- Penne pasta (16 oz.)

What to Do
- Fill a large pot with water and a pinch of salt before placing it

on the stove on top of a burner that has been turned to a high heat. Once the water boils, add in the pasta and let it cook for about 8 minutes until it reaches an al dente state.

- Add the olive oil to a skillet before placing it on top of a burner turned to a high/medium heat. Place the garlic and onion into the skillet and cook until the onion begins to turn tender. Add in the wine along with the tomatoes and let everything cook for 10 minutes, stirring regularly.
- Add in the shrimp and let it cook for 5 minutes. Toss with the pasta and top with parmesan cheese prior to serving.

8: Mediterranean Falafel

This recipe needs 20 minutes to prepare, 20 minutes to cook and will make 4 servings.

- Protein: 11.4 grams
- Carbs: 39.3 grams
- Fats: 9.3 grams
- Calories: 281

What to Use
- Pepper (as desired)
- Extra virgin olive oil (2 T)
- All-purpose flour (1 T)
- Baking soda (.25 T)
- Salt (.25 tsp.)
- Coriander (.25 tsp. ground)
- Cumin (1 tsp. ground)
- Garlic (3 cloves minced)
- Parsley (.25 c chopped)
- Garbanzo beans (15 oz. drained, rinsed)
- Onion (.25 c chopped)

What to Do
- Place the chopped onion into a cheese cloth and squeeze it as hard as possible to remove any excess water.

- Add the baking soda, salt, coriander, cumin, garlic, parsley and garbanzo beans into your food processor and process until the results are becoming pureed but are still somewhat coarse.
- In a mixing bowl, combine the results from the food processor along with the onion and mix well prior to adding in the egg along with the flour. Mix well and shape the results into patties.
- Ensure your oven is set to 400F
- While the oven is warming, add the olive oil to your oven-safe skillet and place it on top of the stove over a burner turner to a high/medium heat. Add the patties to the skillet and let them cook approximately 2.5 minutes per side or until they take on a goldenbrown color.
- Remove the skillet from the stove and place it in the oven. Let the falafel cook approximately 10 minutes or until it is warm all the way through.
- Serve with pita bread and tzatziki and enjoy.

9: Flounder with capers, olives and tomatoes

This recipe needs 20 minutes to prepare, 20 minutes to cook and will make 4servings.

- Protein: 24.4 grams
- Carbs: 8.2 grams
- Fats: 15.4 grams
- Calories: 282

What to Use
- Pepper (as desired)
- Extra virgin olive oil (2 T)
- Basil (6 leaves torn)
- Flounder (1 lb. fillets)
- Parmesan cheese (3 T grated)
- Basil (6 leaves chopped)
- Lemon juice (1 tsp. fresh)
- Capers (.25 c)
- White wine (.25 c)

- Kalamata olives (24 chopped, pitted)
- Italian seasoning (1 pinch)
- Garlic (2 cloves chopped)
- Spanish onion (.5 chopped)
- Tomatoes (5 rinsed)

What to Do

- Ensure your oven is heated to 425F.
- Fill a saucepan with water and a pinch of salt before placing it on the stove on top of a burner that has been turned to a high heat. Once the water boils, add in the tomatoes before pulling them right back out again. Ensure you have a bowl of cold water ready to add them to. Once they are cool enough to handle, remove the skin prior to chopping.
- Add the olive oil to the skillet before placing the skillet on the stove on top of a burner set to a medium heat. Add in the onion and let it cook for about 5 minutes until it is tender. Add in the Italian seasoning, garlic and tomatoes and let everything cook about 6 minutes.
- Add in half of the basil, the lemon juice, capers, wine and olives before turning the heat down and mixing in the parmesan cheese. Let everything cook approximately 15 minutes and it has formed a thick sauce.
- Add the flounder to a baking dish before topping with sauce and basil leaves.
- Place the dish in the oven and let it cook about 10 minutes until the flesh of the fish can easily be flaked with a fork.

10: Costa Brava

This recipe needs 10 minutes to prepare, 25 minutes to cook and will make 10servings.

- Protein: 28.6 grams
- Carbs: 17.6 grams
- Fats: 6.1 grams

- Calories: 239

What to Use

- Pepper (as desired)
- Extra virgin olive oil (2 T)
- Red bell pepper (1 sliced thin)
- Water (2 T)
- Cornstarch (2 T)
- Salsa (.5 c)
- Black olives (2 c)
- Stewed tomatoes (14.5 oz.)
- Yellow onion (1 quartered)
- Garlic (2 cloves minced)
- Cinnamon (1 tsp)
- Cumin (1 tsp)
- Chicken breasts (5 halved)
- Pineapple chunks (20 oz.)

What to Do

- Drain the pineapple but keep the juice. Likely sprinkle salt on top.
- Add the oil to a pan before placing it on the stove on top of a burner turned to a high/medium heat. Add in the chicken before topping with cinnamon and cumin. Mix in the onion and garlic and let everything cook for about 5 minutes.
- Mix in the salsa, olives, tomatoes and pineapple juice. Cover the pan and reduce the heat to allow everything to simmer approximately 25 minutes.
- After the pan has finished simmering, combine the water and cornstarch and add it to the pan juices. Mix in the bell pepper and let the pan simmer until it forms a sauce. Mix in the pineapple chunks and let them simmer until they are warm.
- Top the chicken with the sauce prior to serving.

CONCLUSION

Thank for making it through to the end of this book, let's hope it was informative and able to provide you with all of the tools you need to achieve your goals whatever they may be. The next step is to start using some of these great recipes in your own home. Finally, if you found this book useful in any way, a review on Amazon is always appreciated!

Instant Pot Recipes Cookbook

The Best Instant Pot Recipes for Your Whole Family

CHAPTER 1

WHOLESOME BREAKFAST RECIPES TO GET THE DAY STARTED

Banana French Toast

What's in it

White sugar (1 Tbsp.)
Chopped pecans (4 Tbsp.)
Sliced butter (half a stick)
Cinnamon (.5 tsp.)
Vanilla (1 tsp.)
Milk (.5 c.)
Eggs (3)
Cream cheese (4 Tbsp.)
Brown sugar (2 Tbsp.)
Sliced bananas (4)
Cubed French bread (6 slices)

How's it done

1: Grease a baking dish or use a cake pan. Use a layer of the bread to the bottom and then layer half of the bananas on top.
2: Sprinkle a bit of brown sugar on top and then cover with the cream cheese before topping with the rest of the bread.
3: Add on the other half of the banana slices and sprinkle with some more brown sugar and the pecans. Place the slice dup butter on top.
4: In another bowl, beat the three eggs together before mixing the cinnamon, vanilla, white sugar, and milk inside as well. Pour this on top of the bread to coat.
5: Add some water to your instant pot and situation the steamer basket inside with the dish on top. Secure the lead and seal the pot up.

6: Select Manual and let the timer go for 5 minutes on a high pressure.
7: When this is done, use the quick pressure to release the lid and take it off the pot. Allow the bread to sit for a few minutes before serving.

Apple Oatmeal

What's in it

Chopped walnuts (2 Tbsp.)
Salt (.25 tsp.)
Brown sugar (1 Tbsp.)
Apple cider vinegar (1 tsp.)
Water (2 c.)
Cinnamon (1 tsp.)
Sliced apple (1)
Oats (1 c.)
Butter (2 Tbsp.)

How's it done

1: Select the Saute function on your instant pot and add in a bit of butter to the bottom. Let this melt before adding in the oats and cook for a few minutes.
2: After this time, add in the water, the brown sugar, apple cider vinegar, cinnamon, and apple.
3: Put the lid on securely and seal it all up. Click on manual and let this cook at a higher pressure for about 6 minutes.
4: When the time is up, allow for a natural release of the pressure and then open up the lid.
5: Move all the contents over to the bowl you want to serve in and then top with some walnuts before enjoying.

Breakfast Cobbler

What's in it

Sunflower seeds (2 Tbsp.)
Pecan pieces (.5 c.)
Shredded coconut (.5 c.)
Cinnamon (1 tsp.)
Coconut oil (4 Tbsp.)
Honey (4 Tbsp.)
Diced plums (2)
Diced apples (2)
Diced pears (2)

How's it done

1: Add the cinnamon, coconut oil, honey, diced plums, apples, and pears into the instant pot. Seal up the lid nice and tight.
2: Set this to a high pressure and let the ingredients cook together. After ten minutes, turn off the Instant pot and then use quick pressure release.
3: Open up the lid and then move the fruit over to a bowl, but do not get rid of the liquid.
4: Add in the sunflower seeds, pecans, and coconut to your pot and cook for another five minutes, making sure to stir this around often.
5: When this is done, turn the Instant Pot off and add the seeds over to the prepared fruits before serving.

Egg Bake

What's in it

Chopped green onions
Pepper (.5 tsp.)
Salt (1 tsp.)
Shredded cheddar cheese (.5 c.)
Milk (.25 c.)
Eggs (6)
Hash browns (2 c.)
Sliced mushrooms (1 c.)
Chopped onion (1)
Chopped bacon (6 slices)

How's it done

1: Take out a bowl that is heatproof and will fit into the Instant Pot.
2: Add in the bacon to the Instant Pot and cook to make crispy. Add in the mushrooms and onion and cook a bit before adding in the hash browns to thaw. Turn the Instant pot off.
3: In a bowl, mix the pepper, salt, cheddar cheese, milk, and eggs together. Add in the veggie mixture and the bacon mixture as well.
4: When these are combined, move it all to the bowl you picked out before.
5: Add some water to the Instant Pot before placing the trivet inside and the bowl on top. Secure the lid of the Instant Pot properly.
6: Cook this on a high pressure. After ten minutes are up, turn your Instant Pot off and then release the pressure.
7: Transfer the ingredients inside onto a plate and garnish with the green onions before serving.

Egg Muffins

What's in it

Chopped green onion (1)
Crumbled bacon (4 slices)
Shredded cheddar (4 Tbsp.)
Lemon pepper seasoning (.25 tsp.)
Eggs (4)

How's it done

1: Add a bit of water to your Instant Pot along with a steamer basket.
2: Take out a bowl and beat the eggs with the lemon pepper seasoning.
Divide the green onion, bacon, and cheese between four muffin cups.
3: Add the eggs on top of the cups and then stir around a bit before adding into the Instant Pot.
4: Secure the lid well and then let this cook on a high pressure. After eight minutes are up, turn the pressure cooker off and give it some time for the pressure to release.
5: Take the lid off the Instant Pot and then take the muffin cups out to serve.

Sausage Frittata

What's in it

Pepper
Salt
Cooked sausage (.5 c.)
Cheddar cheese (4 Tbsp.)
Sour cream (2 Tbsp.)
Beaten eggs (4)
Water (2 c.)

Coconut oil (1 Tbsp.)

How's it done

1: Use a bit of coconut oil to grease up a baking dish. Add the water to the Instant Pot and then add in a steam basket as well.
2: Whisk together the sour cream and the eggs until well combined. Then stir in the pepper, salt, sausage, and cheese. Stir before pouring into the baking dish.
3: Use some foil to cover up the dish and then place inside of the Instant Pot. Close the lid and let this cook on a low pressure.
4: After 20 minutes, use a quick release pressure before opening up the Instant Pot. Top this dish with some more cheese before serving.

Tomato and Spinach Quiche

What's in it

Parmesan cheese (4 Tbsp.)
Tomato slices (4)
Chopped green onions (2)
Diced tomatoes (.5 c.)
Spinach (1.5 c.)
Pepper
Salt
Milk (.25 c.)
Eggs (6)

How's it done

1: Add a trivet to the bottom of your Instant Pot along with some water.
2: In a bowl, whisk together the pepper, salt, milk, and eggs until well combined.

3: Take out a baking dish and add in the green onions, tomatoes, and spinach to mix well. Top with your egg mixture and then place the sliced tomatoes on top with some Parmesan cheese.

4: Place the prepared baking dish on the trivet in the Instant Pot. Turn this on a high pressure.

5: After twenty minutes, turn the Instant Pot off and let the pressure release a bit. Open the lid and take the baking dish out before serving.

CHAPTER 2

LUNCH RECIPES TO HELP KEEP YOU FULL

Vegetable and Beef Soup

What's in it

Oregano (.5 tsp.)
Parsley (2 tsp.)
Pepper
Salt
Tomato paste (3 Tbsp.)
Cubed potatoes (2)
Sliced celery (3)
Sliced carrots (4)
Stewed tomatoes (1 can)
Minced garlic cloves (4)
Diced onion (1)
Beef (2 lbs.)

How's it done

1: Turn on the Instant Pot to Saute. Add in the garlic, onion, and ground beef and keep cooking until the beef is browned. When it is done, drain off the grease.

2: Add in the stewed tomatoes and cook a bit longer.

3: After a few minutes add in the rest of the ingredients and then place the lid on top. Cook at a high pressure.

4: After four minutes are up, use the quick release method to get rid of the pressure. Move the soup over to some serving bowls before enjoying.

Chicken Noodle

What's in it

Parsley (4 Tbsp.)
Egg noodles (4 oz.)
Pepper (.5 tsp.)
Water (8 c.)
Soy sauce (2 Tbsp.)
Whole chicken (1)
Sliced celery (2)
Carrots (4)
Minced garlic cloves (4)
Diced onion (1)
Olive oil (1 Tbsp.)

How's it done

1: To preheat the Instant Pot, turn it on to Saute and then add in the olive oil. When this is hot, cook the onion for a bit and add in the celery, carrots, and garlic.
2: Add the chicken into the Instant Pot as well as the pepper, salt, soy sauce, water. Place the lid on top and seal the lid.
3: Cook this on a high pressure. After twenty minutes, quickly release the pressure and open the lid. Take the chicken out and shred it up.
4: Turn the heat back on with the Instant Pot and let this broth come to a boil. Add in the egg noodles and let them cook until soft.
5: Shred up the chicken into smaller pieces, getting rid of the skin and bone. Stir it back into the broth.
6: Adjust the seasonings how you would like and enjoy.

Cheesy Potato Soup

What's in it

Corn (1 c.)
Half and half (2 c.)
Shredded cheese (1 c.)
Cubed cream cheese (3 oz.)
Cornstarch mixed with water (2 Tbsp. each)
Parsley (2 Tbsp.)
Pepper
Salt
Chicken broth (2 c.)
Cubed potatoes (4)
Chopped onion (1)
Butter (2 Tbsp.)
Crumbled bacon (6 slices)

How's it done

1: Take out the Instant Pot and turn it on. Heat up the butter and once it is melted, add in the chopped onion, cooking to make tender.

2: At this time, add the parsley, pepper, salt, and half the chicken broth. Add the steamer basket inside and add the potatoes to the basket.

3: Place the lid on the Instant Pot and cook on a high pressure. After five minutes, release the pressure naturally and take the steamer basket out.

4: Add in the cornstarch and water mixture and stir around. Add the cheddar cheese, cream cheese, corn, bacon, cooked potatoes, half and half and the rest of the chicken broth.

4: Heat this all up so that it comes to a boil. Turn the Instant Pot off and transfer this over to serving bowls before enjoying.

Chicken Tacos

What's in it

Taco seasoning (1 Tbsp.)
Salsa (1 c.)
Water (.5 c.)
Chicken breasts (3)

How's it done

1: Place the chicken inside of your Instant Pot along with the taco seasoning, salsa, and water.
2: Place the lid on top of the Instant Pot and let it cook on a high pressure. After fifteen minutes and then use quick pressure release to let it all out.
3: Take the lid off the Instant Pot and then shred the chicken with two forks and stir it around. Add to your favorite shells or to some lettuce and serve.

General Tso's Chicken

What's in it

Sesame seeds (1 Tbsp.)
Cornstarch (2 Tbsp.)
Minced garlic cloves (2)
Grated ginger (.25 tsp.)
Red pepper flakes (.25 tsp.)
Hoisin sauce (3 Tbsp.)
Brown sugar (4 Tbsp.)
Soy sauce (4 Tbsp.)
Rice vinegar (6 Tbsp.)
Sesame oil (1 tsp.)
Cubed chicken (1.5 lbs.)
White rice, cooked (2 c.)
Chopped green onion (1)

How's it done

1: Turn on the Instant Pot and add in the sesame oil. Add in the chicken and let it cook for a few minutes.
2: While that is cooking, add together the garlic cloves, ginger, pepper flakes, hoisin sauce, brown sugar, soy sauce, and rice vinegar. Pour this over the chicken in the Instant Pot.
3: Add the lid to the pot and cook the chicken on a high pressure. After ten minutes, allow the pressure to quickly release from the pot.
4: Once you take the lid off, whisk the cornstarch inside and let it cook a bit longer.
5: Before serving, garnish with some green onions and sesame seeds and enjoy.

Spicy Moroccan Chicken

What's in it

Chicken stock (.5 c.)
Black pepper
Salt (1 tsp.)
Butter (1 Tbsp.)
Coriander (.25 tsp.)
Cinnamon (.5 tsp.)
Ginger (.5 tsp.)
Cumin (1 tsp.)
Garlic powder (1 tsp.)
Paprika (1 tsp.)
Chicken drumsticks (1 lb.)
Lemon zest (1 tsp.)
Lemon juice (1 Tbsp.)
Blackstrap molasses (2 tsp.)
Honey (4 Tbsp.)

How's it done

1: Take out a bowl and mix together the coriander, cinnamon, ginger, cumin, garlic powder, and paprika.
2: Using some towels, dry the chicken and then coat with the spices all over.
3: Turn on the Instant Pot and add in some butter. Place the chicken inside and brown it on all sides for about ten minutes.
4: Add in half a cup of the chicken stock. Secure the lid and then let this cook on a high pressure.
5: After ten minutes, you can turn the Instant Pot off and let the pressure out. move the chicken over to a bowl.
6: Mix together the lemon zest, lemon juice, molasses, and honey. Pour this into the Instant Pot and cook, without the lid on, for a bit longer to make it thick.
7: Use this sauce to coat your chicken. Serve with some green onions on top.

Beef Stroganoff

What's in it

Chopped white onion (1)
Sliced mushrooms (2 c.)
Olive oil (2 Tbsp.)
Cubed sirloin tip roast (2 lbs.)
Paprika (.25 tsp.)
Thyme (.5 tsp.)
Rosemary (.5 tsp.)
Garlic powder (.25 tsp.)
Onion powder (.25 tsp.)
Pepper (.5 tsp.)
Salt (.75 tsp.)
Flour (.75 c.)
Sour cream (.75 c.)

Beef broth (1.5 c.)
Minced garlic cloves (2)

How's it done

1: To get started, mix together the paprika, rosemary, thyme, garlic powder, onion powder, pepper, salt, and flour together. Add in the beef and toss it around to coat.

2: Turn on the Instant Pot and heat up some olive oil. Once this is hot, add in the prepared beef and brown it on all sides. You may need to do this in batches.

3: Add in the onions and mushrooms and cook before needing to add in the garlic.

4: Move the meet back to the Instant Pot along with the beef broth. Place the lid on the Instant Pot and cook at a high pressure.

5: After twenty minutes are up, turn off the Instant Pot and let the pressure naturally release.

6: Take the lid off and stir in the sour cream. Add some pepper and salt before serving over egg noodles.

Smoked Brisket

What's in it

Thyme (1 Tbsp.)
Liquid smoke (1 Tbsp.)
Chicken stock (2 c.)
Smoked paprika (.5 tsp.)
Onion powder (1 tsp.)
Mustard powder (1 tsp.)
Pepper (1 tsp.)
Salt (2 tsp.)
Maple sugar (2 Tbsp.)
Beef brisket (1.5 lbs.)

How's it done

1: Pat the brisket dry with a paper towel. Taking out a bowl mix the paprika, onion powder, mustard powder, pepper, salt, and maple sugar together. Use this to coat the meat all over.

2: Turn the Instant Pot on and grease it with some cooking oil. Add in the brisket and brown until it is golden and then flip it over.

3: Add the thyme, liquid smoke, and stock. Place the lid on top and cook at a high pressure.

4: After fifty minutes are done, take the pressure out and then take the lid off. Remove the brisket with some tongs and then cover with a bit of foil.

5: Let the sauces in the Instant Pot cook for a bit longer so that the sauce can thicken, keeping the lid off.

6: Slice up the brisket and then serve with the sauce and the veggies of your choices.

Instant Pot Hamburger Helper

What's in it

American cheese (4 oz.)
Cheddar cheese (16 oz.)
Heavy cream (8 o.)
Elbow macaroni (16 oz.)
Beef broth (2 c.)
Garlic powder (1 Tbsp.)
Onion powder (1 Tbsp.)
Ground beef (1 lb.)

How's it done

1: Turn on the Instant Pot to heat up a bit and add in the garlic powder, onion powder, and ground beef. Cook while crumbling up the meat and it is no longer pink.

2: Add in some heavy cream, the macaroni, and beef broth. Place the lid on the Instant Pot and cook on a high pressure.
3: After five minutes, turn the Instant Pot off and let the pressure slowly release.
4: Open up the lid and add in the American cheese and the cheddar cheese before serving.

Spiced Chicken Wrap

What's in it

Ground mustard (1 tsp.)
Ground cumin (1 tsp.)
Apple cider vinegar (3 Tbsp.)
Coconut oil (4 Tbsp.)
Chicken breast (1 lb.)
Romaine lettuce leaves (6)
Pepper (1 tsp.)
Paprika (1 tsp.)

How's it done

1: Take out a bowl and combine together the pepper, paprika, mustard, cumin, coconut oil, and apple cider vinegar.
2: Rub your chicken with some of the vinegar mixture, some oil, and the spice mixture and then let it marinate for half an hour or more.
3: When read, turn the Instant Pot on and add in the rest of the oil along with the chicken breasts. Cook long enough to brown.
4: Add in two cups of water to the pressure cooker and then turn to a high pressure. After twenty minutes, take the chicken out of the cooker and shred it up.
5: Take a piece of the lettuce and scoop some of the chicken on top. Sprinkle on the leftover vinegar and spices and then wrap it up.

6: Repeat the steps with the rest of the leaves and the chicken before serving.

Bacon and Chicken Meal

What's in it

Whipping cream (.5 c.)
Coconut oil (4 Tbsp.)
Bacon (.5 lb.)
Chicken breast fillet (1 lb.)
Prepared mustard (2 Tbsp.)
Butter (3 Tbsp.)

How's it done

1: To start, slice up the chicken breast into smaller pieces and then wrap each part with a slice of bacon.
2: Spray a baking pan with some cooking spray and then place the bacon wrapped chicken into the pan.
3: Take out the Instant Pot and turn it on. Add the oil and let it heat up before adding the bacon and chicken until they are browned.
4: While those are cooking, you can make the dipping sauce. To do this, melt the butter on the stove and whisk in the cream. Heat for a minute.
5: When this is warm, take it off the heat and add the mustard. Serve it with the bacon wrapped chicken and have a favorite side.

Cheesy Hotdog Huggers

What's in it
Cheddar cheese (2 o.)
Bacon (1 lb.)
Hot dogs (1 lb.)
Pepper
Salt
Onion powder (1 tsp.)
Garlic powder (1 tsp.)

How's it done

1: Turn on your pressure cooker to a high setting and add in two cups of water. Score the hotdogs with a slit going lengthwise.

2: Slice up your cheese into strips that are the length of your hotdogs and then insert them inside.

3: Wrap a slice of bacon around each hot dog and then seal with a wooden pick. Place these into the steamer basket inside the Instant Pot.

4: Place the lid onto the Instant Pot and seal it up. After about five minutes, quickly release the pressure and then enjoy.

CHAPTER 3

SNACKS FOR THE MIDDLE OF THE DAY

BBQ Chicken Drumsticks

What's in it

Pepper
Salt
Minced garlic cloves (2)
BBQ sauce (2 c.)
Chili sauce (.25 c.)
Honey (3 Tbsp.)
Chicken drumsticks (1.5 lbs.)

How's it done

1: Take out the Instant Pot and turn it on. Add the pepper, salt, garlic cloves, BBQ sauce, chili sauce, honey, and chicken.
2: Close the lid and set to a low pressure. Cook this for about 2 hours.
3: Slowly release the pressure over a few minutes before taking the chicken out and serving.

Cocktail Meatballs

What's in it

Apple or grape jelly (1 c.)
Cocktail or chili sauce (.5 c.)
Meatballs (24 oz.)

How's it done

1: Turn on your Instant Pot to heat up. While this is heating up, mix together the chili sauce and the jelly.

2: Place your meatballs into the prepared Instant Pot and pour the jelly mixture on top.
3: Place the lid on top of the meatballs and cook at a high pressure.
4: After five minutes, turn the Instant Pot off and slowly release the pressure. Take the meatballs off and then let the sauce simmer a few more minutes.
5: Insert some toothpicks before serving.

Blue Cheese Beets

What's in it

Water (1 c.)
Crumbled blue cheese (.25 c.)
Pepper
Salt
Beets (6)

How's it done

1: Place the beets into the Instant Pot steamer basket. Add in a cup of water and cook on a high pressure.
2: After twenty minutes, let the pressure release naturally and remove the beets. When they have cooled down a bit before slicing into quarters.
3: Place the beets into a bowl with the pepper, salt, and blue cheese. Stir these together before serving.

Tomato Salad

What's in it

Pecans (2 oz.)
Cherry tomatoes (1 pint)
Sugar (2 Tbsp.)
Pepper

Salt
Pickling juice (2 tsp.)
Water (1 c.)
Apple cider vinegar (1 c.)
Goat cheese (4 oz.)
Sliced red onion (1)
Trimmed beets (8)
Water (1.5 c.)
Olive oil (2 Tbsp.)

How's it done

1: Put the beets into a steamer basket into the Instant Pot and add in the water. Place the water inside and then cook at a high pressure.

2: After twenty minutes, release the pressure and move the beets to a cutting board. Let these cool down a bit before peeling and chopping them out.

3: Clean out the Instant Pot and add in another cup of water along with the salt, pickling juice, sugar, and vinegar.

4: Cover the Instant Pot and let these ingredients on a high setting for another two minutes.

5: Release the pressure and strain out the liquid into a bowl. Add in the onions and lave alone for a few minutes.

6: Add the beets and the tomatoes and stir around. Add the pepper, salt, and olive oil and top with the pecans and goat cheese before serving.

Stuffed Bell Peppers

What's in it

Bell peppers, without tops or seeds (4)
Salt
Cumin (1 tsp.)
Garlic powder (1 tsp.)

Panko (1 c.)
Chili powder (2 tsp.)
Chopped jalapeno pepper (1)
Chopped green chilies (5 oz.)
Chopped green onions (2)
Water (1 c.)
Ground turkey (1 lb.)
Pico de gallo
Tortilla chips
Chopped avocado (1)
Pepper Jack cheese (4 slices)
Chipotle Sauce
Garlic powder (.25 tsp.)
Chipotle in adobo sauce (2 Tbsp.)
Sour cream (.5 c.)
Juice from a lime (1)

How's it done

1: Take out a bowl and mix together the garlic powder, lime juice, lime zest, chipotle in adobo sauce, and sour cream. Keep it in the fridge for a bit.

2: In another bowl, mix the garlic powder, chili powder, salt, cumin, jalapeno, bread crumbs, green chilies, green onions, and turkey.

3: When the second mixture is done, use it to stuff the prepared peppers.

4: Add some water to the heating up Instant Pot and then add the peppers to the steamer basket.

5: Cover the Instant Pot and cook on a high setting. After fifteen minutes, let the pressure release naturally for ten minutes and move the bell peppers to a pan.

6: Add the cheese on top and then place under the broiler until the cheese is browned.

7: Divide up the peppers and then top with the chipotle sauce and enjoy.

Tasty Sweet Carrots

What's in it

Water (.5 c.)
Butter (.5 Tbsp.)
Brown sugar (1 Tbsp.)
Salt
Baby carrots (2 c.)

How's it done

1: Take out the Instant Pot and mix together the sugar, salt, water, and
butter inside. Turn the Instant Pot on and let these melt together.
2: Add in the carrots, stir things together and then cover the Instant Pot.
Cook these ingredients on high.
3: After fifteen minutes have passed, release the pressure and take the
list off. Let everything cook for a bit longer and then serve.

Cabbage and Sausage

What's in it

Chopped tomatoes, canned (15 oz.)
Sliced sausage links (1 lb.)
Pepper
Salt
Chopped cabbage head (1)
Butter (3)
Turmeric (2 tsp.)
Chopped yellow onion (.5 c.)

How's it done

1: Set the Instant Pot so that it starts to warm up and then add in the slices of sausage. Cook these until they become brown.

2: Drain out any grease that is leftover before adding in the turmeric, onion, pepper, tomatoes, salt, cabbage, and butter.

3: Place the lid on top of the Instant Pot and then cook on a high pressure.

4: After two minutes have passed, do a quick release of the pressure and then uncover the pot.

5: Divide up the sausage and cabbage before serving.

Eggplant Delight

What's in it

Pepper
Salt
Garlic powder (1 Tbsp.)
Minced garlic cloves (3)
Olive oil (1 Tbsp.)
Cubed eggplant (4 c.)
Water (.5 c.)
Marinara sauce (1 c.)

How's it done

1: To start this recipe, set the Instant Pot to heat up and add in the oil and the garlic. Cook for a few minutes.

2: Now add in the water, marinara sauce, garlic powder, pepper, salt, and eggplant. Place the lid on top and cook this at a high pressure.

3: After about 8 minutes, use the quick release method to let the pressure out and take the lid off.

4: Serve this eggplant mixture on its own or with some noodles for a great dinner.

CHAPTER 4

DELICIOUS DESSERTS YOU ARE GOING TO LOVE

Banana Bread

What's in it

Baking powder (1 tsp.)
Mashed bananas (2)
Egg (1)
Vanilla (1 tsp.)
Soft ghee (.3 c.)
Coconut sugar (.75 c.)
Cooking spray
Water (2 c.)
Cream of tartar (1.5 tsp.)
Cashew milk (.3 c.)
Baking soda (.5 tsp.)
Salt
Flour (1.5 c.)

How's it done

1: Take out a bowl and mix together the cream of tartar and the milk. When those are combined, add in the bananas, vanilla, egg, ghee, and sugar.
2: In another bowl, mix the baking soda, baking powder, salt, and flour.
3: Now combine both of these mixtures and then pour it into the cake pan. Place the steamer basket into your instant pot and place the baking pan inside as well.
4: Add some water to your Instant Pot and then put the lid on top. Cook at a high pressure.

5: After thirty minutes, release the pressure and then take the lid off. Take the bread out of the Instant Pot and then let it cool down a bit before serving.

Apple Crisp

What's in it

Water (.5 c.)
Maple syrup (1 Tbsp.)
Nutmeg (.5 tsp.)
Chopped apples (5)
Cinnamon (2 tsp.)
Salt
Sugar (.25 c.)
Rolled oats (.75 c.)
Flour (.25 c.)
Butter (4 Tbsp.)

How's it done

1: Place your apples into the Instant Pot. Add in the water, maple syrup, nutmeg, and cinnamon.
2: In a separate bowl, mix the flour, salt, sugar, oats, and butter and stir well.
3: Drop some of this mixture on top of the apples and place the lid on top. Cook on a high pressure.
4: After eight minutes are up, let the pressure out and then serve this warm.

Chocolate and Pumpkin Cake

What's in it

Pumpkin pie spice (.75 tsp.)
Baking soda (1 tsp.)
Salt
Whole wheat flour (.75 c.)
White flour (.75 c.)
Chocolate chips (.6 c.)
Vanilla (.5 tsp.
Egg (1)
Water (1 quart)
Cooking spray
Pumpkin puree, canned (8 o.)
Greek yogurt (.5 c.)
Canola oil (2 Tbsp.)
Baking powder (.5 tsp.)
Mashed banana (1)
Sugar (.75 c.)

How's it done

1: Take out a bowl and mix together the pumpkin spice, baking powder, baking soda, salt, whole wheat flour, and white flour and stir it well.
2: Take out the second bowl and use a mixer to combine the banana, oil, sugar, egg, vanilla, pumpkin puree, and yogurt.
3: When these are both done, combine together your two mixtures, adding in the chocolate chips as you go.
4: Pour all of the ingredients into a Bundt pan and cover with some paper towels and foil. Place the steamer basket into the Instant Pot and add the Bundt pan.
5: Add some water to the pot and place the lid on top. Cook this at a high pressure.

6: After 35 minutes, start slow releasing the pressure and then take the lid off. Allow the cake some time to cool down before you slice it up and serve.

Holiday Pudding

What's in it

Chopped apricots, dried (4 oz.)
Water (2 c.)
Olive oil (1 Tbsp.)
Dried cranberries (4 oz.)
Grated carrot (1)
Eggs (4)
Maple syrup (3 Tbsp.)
Butter (15 Tbsp.)
Salt
Cinnamon powder
Ginger powder (1 tsp.)
Sugar (1 c.)
Baking powder (3 tsp.)
White flour (1 c.)

How's it done

1: Grease a pudding mold with some oil and then set to the side.
2: Take out your blender and pulse together the ginger, salt, cinnamon, sugar, baking powder, and flour.
3: Add the butter, eggs, and maple syrup and pulse in between each thing. Now add in the carrot and the dried fruits and let them fold into the batter.
4: Spread out this mix into a pudding mold and then add the steamer basket and two cups of water into your Instant Pot.
5: Place the pudding mold into the Instant Pot and then place the lid on top. Steam the pudding on a high pressure.

6: After 30 minutes, slowly release the pressure and then take it out to cool down a bit before serving.

Apple Cake

What's in it

Sugar (.25 c.)
Ricotta cheese (1 c.)
Water (2 c.)
Chopped apple (1)
Sliced apple (1)
Baking soda (1 tsp.)
Cinnamon powder (.25 tsp.)
Baking powder (2 tsp.)
White flour (1 c.)
Olive oil (3 Tbsp.)
Vanilla (1 tsp.)
Egg (1)
Lemon juice (1 Tbsp.)

How's it done

1: Bring out a bowl and add the sliced and chopped apples along with the lemon juice together before leaving to the side.
2: Take out a dish and line with some parchment paper. Add in some oil and dust with flour. Sprinkle the sugar on the bottom and arrange your sliced apples on top of it.
3: In another bowl, mix together the oil, vanilla, sugar, cheese, and egg and stir well. Add in the cinnamon, baking soda, baking powder, and flour as well.
4: Now add the chopped apple, toss around, and then pour it into the prepared pan.
5: Add a steamer basket to the Instant Pot and some water. Place the pan into the Instant Pot and cook at a high pressure.

6: After 20 minutes, let the pressure release, take the lid off the pot, and then serve the cake.

Pumpkin Pie

What's in it

Maple syrup (.75 c.)
Whole milk (1 c.)
Water (2 c.)
Eggs (2)
Chopped butternut squash (2 lbs.)
Chopped pecans
Whipped cream
Cornstarch (1 Tbsp.)
Salt
Powdered cloves (.25 tsp.)
Powdered ginger (.5 tsp.)
Cinnamon powder (1 tsp.)

How's it done

1: To start this recipe, place the cubes of squash into a steamer basket and then place into the Instant Pot. Add in some water and place the lid on top.
2: Cook these on a high pressure. After four minutes are up, turn the Instant Pot off and then release the pressure, moving the squash over to a strainer to cool down.
3: Mash up the squash a bit inside a bowl before adding the cloves, salt, ginger, cinnamon, eggs, milk, and maple syrup to it.
4: Pour this mixture into some ramekins and then into the steamer basket again. Add in some more water to the pot and cover it up, cooking at a high pressure.
5: After ten minutes, release the pressure and take the ramekins out.

After they have some time to cool down, top with whipped cream and pecans before serving.

CONCLUSION

Thank for making it through to the end of this book, let's hope it was informative and able to provide you with all of the tools you need to achieve your goals whatever they may be.

The next step is to take out your Instant Pot and start using some of these great recipes in your own home. The Instant Pot is not just a great way to make meals quickly, it can be a great way to eat foods that are healthy and wholesome for you. This guidebook contained all of the great recipes that you need to eat healthily and get all the benefits that come from using the Instant Pot. So the next time you are looking for a tasty meal for your family, something good to fill you up in the morning, or even a good dessert everyone will love, make sure to pull out this guidebook and see just how great the Instant Pot can be, not only to save you time, but to help you eat healthy.

Finally, if you found this book useful in any way, a review on Amazon is always appreciated!

The Complete Guide to Intermittent Fasting

Learn Everything You Need About Intermittent Fasting and All the Benefits Associated with It

INTRODUCTION

The following chapters will discuss everything you need to know about intermittent fasting, what it is and what are the different types. You will also learn about the history of fasting, how it actually feels when you fast, and what the benefits and drawbacks are.

Man has been fasting from time immemorial. From the days of ancient Egypt to Palestine and communities around the world, fasting has been around for centuries. People fast for different reasons. A majority of them wish to lose weight. Others do it for religious reasons while many others do it for health reasons.

Whatever your reasons for fasting are, this book will teach you how to do it the right way, which methods work and how to stay the course and put up with the challenges that may come your way. If you are able to focus on the benefits of fasting and take things one step at a time, then you will emerge victorious and you will enjoy the benefits of fasting while avoiding the drawbacks.

Fasting is an important aspect of life that millions of people undertake each day. You, too, can benefit from the positive effects of fasting. By reading this book, you will get the information you need to fast effectively and continue fasting for as long as you wish.

There are plenty of books on this subject on the market, thanks again for choosing this one! Every effort was made to ensure it is full of as much useful information as possible, please enjoy!

CHAPTER 1

WHY IS FASTING ACTUALLY GOOD FOR HEALTH?

What is fasting?

Fasting is simply going without drink or food for a period of time. People fast for a variety of reasons. Some fast to observe religious obligations while others do so to cleanse their bodies. People also fast in order to lose weight and for other reasons too.

There are different types of fasting. For instance, normal fasting is abstinence from food and drink, except water. Dry fasting is where you abstain from all food and drink, including water, for a given period of time.

Intermittent fasting

The term intermittent fasting is a type of fasting with periods where you eat and drink and other periods where you fast. It can also be described as a cycle between periods of fasting and periods of regular food intakes.

Intermittent fasting focuses more on when you should eat but not necessarily what foods you should eat. This is why there are different types of intermittent fasting methods. Each method splits a single day or a whole week into periods of fasting and periods when you are allowed to eat.

Intermittent fasting can be as simple as skipping breakfast. Suppose you go to bed at 9.00 pm and sleep. You then wake up by 7 and have your first meal at 12.00 noon, skipping breakfast altogether. This can be considered a type of intermittent fasting. It has many benefits to your body, mind and overall health and wellbeing. It is broadly divided into three broad categories.

ADF – Alternate Day Fasting: This is a type of intermittent fasting which starts with a 24-hour fast that is followed by a 24-hour non-fasting period. In this type of fast, you can choose to fast for 23 hours and then have a single meal before the day is over.

TRF – Time Restricted Fasting: In this type of fasting, you will fast for a couple of hours each day and then set aside a few hours within which you can eat. For instance, you can fast for 16 hours each day and then eat your daily calorie requirements within the remaining 8 hours.

Whole-day Fasting: This type of fasting includes some fasting and some non-fasting days. It can be expressed as a ratio such as 5:2. During fasting days, you may eat only 400-500 calories if you are female and 500-600 for males. On non-fasting days, you can eat normally.

Reasons why fasting is actually good for your health

1. Fasting can help you lose weight, including belly fat

One of the best ways to lose weight and keep it off is through fasting. Intermittent fasting will cause you to eat fewer meals each day. This means your calories intake will reduce. If you do this regularly, then you will definitely lose weight.

Hormonal functions are enhanced when you fast which also facilitates weight loss. Some of these include increased growth hormone levels, lower insulin amounts as well as a rise in the levels of noradrenaline. All these will result in faster breakdown of body fat and this fat is then broken down and expended as energy.

2. Intermittent fasting can help reduce insulin resistance

Type 2 diabetes has become endemic around the world. It affects millions of people of all demographics. The main feature of type

II diabetes is high blood sugar levels due to insulin resistance by the body. Intermittent fasting has been shown to reduce insulin resistance which helps in the management of type II diabetes.

3. Intermittent fasting is beneficial for the health of your heart

Did you know that heart disease is the currently the biggest killer? And there are certain risk factors, also known as health markers that are associated with increased or decreased risk of heart health. Fasting helps to improve these markers. For instance, it helps lower blood pressure, lowers blood sugar, bad cholesterol, and even inflammatory markers.

4. It may help to prevent cancer

Cancer is a terrible disease and now affects more people than ever before. It manifests by abnormal growth of cells. The positive effects of intermittent fasting on cancer may help reduce the risk of cancer.

There are many other benefits of fasting. For instance, fasting is good for the brain. It helps build strong and lean muscle, prevents debilitating diseases such as Alzheimer's disease and extends lifespan, helping people live longer.

CHAPTER 2

WHO CAN BENEFIT FROM FASTING?

Fasting has been determined to provide many health benefits. These benefits can be traced back to the days of Hippocrates. They extend into almost every sphere of our lives. These include weight management, development of lean muscles, good cardiovascular health and many others.

Different kinds of people are set to benefit from fasting. For instance, intermittent fasting may help someone with health issues. Studies carried out on animals show great promise on health and other numerous benefits as well. There is also irrefutable evidence which indicates that timed periods of fasting are great for our overall health and wellbeing.

So, who can benefit from fasting?

1: Anyone who is overweight or obese

Carrying around excess weight is dangerous for your health and well-being. It can be the cause of cardiovascular diseases and conditions such as high blood pressure and diabetes. Excessive body weight also affects mobility, self-esteem, appearance and other aspects of our lives.

Fasting is a great and safe way of losing weight. It allows the body to use its own fat reserves as a source of energy. This loosens up and burns fat that is stored in the body. By losing weight, you will decrease your risk of cardiovascular diseases and some chronic conditions, you will look and feel better and with overall be healthier.

2: People at risk of, or suffering from, type II diabetes

Diabetes is a serious chronic condition that affects millions of people around the world. Fasting improves body's sensitivity to insulin so it can better handle blood sugar. After a period of fasting, studies indicate that insulin effectiveness in the body becomes more effective.

3: Health and fitness enthusiasts

If you love keeping fit, working out and being in great form, then fasting is one of the ways that can help you achieve this. By fasting, you lose weight and with reduced body mass, you will develop strong, lean muscles and enable you to work harder. Fasting is great for athletes, fitness enthusiasts and anyone serious about sports.

4: People suffering from high blood pressure

Fasting can significantly lower blood pressure. Many people who fast record lower blood pressure. This is not necessarily caused directly by fasting but by reduced salt intake as well as loss of salt in the blood through urine and sweating.

5: Any person at risk of cardiovascular disease

Heart and cardiovascular diseases have become very common and are the number one killer. Anyone at risk of cardiovascular diseases should consider fasting in order to improve their health. By fasting, the cardiovascular system loses fat and arteries get unclogged. The heart starts beating normally again which leads to an overall better cardio system. There are credible reports of patients with heart conditions who have seen tremendous health improvement after they began to fast.

6: Stressed, anxious and depressed people

Another group of people that would definitely benefit from fasting are those with mental health problems such as anxiety or stress. These conditions are a lot more common than people think. Fasting causes blood to flow better with better blood composition, healthier gene signaling and improved hormone signaling. All these will help improve your mental health condition.

Many other people can benefit from fasting. They include those who want to maintain their youthful good looks and live stress-free lives, anyone who wants to maintain a healthy brain, those who wish to have healthy skin and so many others.

Any person facing mobility challenges due to weight-related issues should also consider fasting. However, those with any major medical condition should consult a doctor before they begin to fast.

Intermittent fasting summary

There is no intake of calories during fasting. All food is to be taken once the fast is over. However, zero-calorie drinks such as water, coffee and tea are allowed. Food choice still matters but meal frequency does not.

A large part of your fast is spent during sleep. Your meals will vary on days when you have to work out. The best way to fast is to find a method that suits your lifestyle and one that you are comfortable with.

CHAPTER 3

THE HISTORY OF FASTING

Fasting is described as willful abstinence from some or all food and drink for a period of time. The idea of fasting has been around for ages and is as old as mankind. There is no period in history when man did not fast.

All written records and all other sources of information regardless of origin, territory, religion, or race, mentions fasting as an integral part of humanity. This shows that fasting had been part of humanity and has been recognized for its benefits and effectiveness.

Ancient philosophers and thinkers recognized fasting

According to Greek historian Herodotus who lived between 484 and 425 BC, the Egyptians were the healthiest people on earth. He observed that for three days each month, they would purify their bodies by performing enemas and vomiting. Egyptians apparently believed that all illnesses emanated from the food we eat.

Even Hippocrates, a great physician and the father of modern medicine, was a great believer in moderation and ardent supporter of treatment through fasting. He believed that when a man is fed, the disease is fed too.

Many other philosophers, healers, and thinkers all believed in fasting. They used it as a healing therapy and a means to good health. They include Plato, Socrates, Galen, and Aristotle.

Religious and cultural reasons

Fasting was recognized by religions. In the Holy Bible, for instance, there are over 30 references to fasting. There are also numerous instances where fasting is referenced among other religious groups. Fasting has, as a religious observance, been practiced for many centuries. Its practice is believed to even surpass even recorded history.

In many primitive cultures, fasting was required before important events such as war or coming-of-age rituals. The purpose back then was to pacify perhaps an angry deity and also as a rite to prevent or avoid calamities such as famine, disease and so on.

Other religions, apart from Christianity, embraced fasting as well. For instance, Judaism and Islam still embrace fasting to this day, something that they have been practicing for centuries. Judaism observes some annual fasting days such as the Day of Atonement or Yom Kippur. Muslims, on the other hand, observe fasting during the holy month of Ramadan. Eastern Orthodox and Roman Catholics fast to observe special occasions such as Lent, the 40-day period when Jesus fasted. In other religions, fasting was and is still used as a means of communicating with a deity. For instance, the gods were thought to reveal important teachings in visions and dreams only after priests participate in a meaningful fast.

Political protests

Fasting has long been used as a political tool, especially by political prisoners. Famous politicians such as Mahatma Gandhi and the Suffragettes effectively used fasting as a tool to express their opinions. Mahatma Gandhi is considered the father of modern India.

In his non-violent campaigns, he used fasting effectively to express his points. During the struggle for India's independence, he used hunger strikes as a means of non-violent resistance. He fasted at least 17 times, the longest of which lasted 21 days. Still, in India, Jatin Das, who was agitating for the independence of the country, fasted to death. He had fasted for 116 days continuously.

His counterparts in the fast, Bhagat Singh and Dutt, gave up after surpassing the current world record of 97 days which was set by an Irishman.

Therapeutic fasting

People have been fasting for many centuries for many other purposes. Therapeutic fasting is one of the reasons. People back then used fasting to treat or prevent diseases. Therapeutic fasting became popular in the 19th century and formed part of the Natural Hygiene Movement in the United States. This movement focused on preventing ill health through fasting but under medical supervision.

The pioneer of therapeutic fasting in America is Dr. Herbert Shelton. According to him, he assisted over 40,000 patients to recover through fasting after suffering serious medical conditions. Even in the UK, fasting has for many years been used for purposes of health, wellbeing and for treating illnesses. Fasting was very popular in the 1920s when the emphasis was on diet, exercise, fresh air, positive thinking, sunshine, and fasting.

As part of treatment, fasting was commonly adopted to treat high blood pressure, digestive problems, heart disease, obesity, headaches, allergies and a lot of other conditions. Therapeutic fasts are not standard but are tailored to suit individual needs depending on what is being treated and other factors.

Today, fasting remains relevant in our lives. It is applied in many different situations and for different purposes by different people. There is sufficient proof that fasting is definitely good for us and has numerous benefits when properly exercised.

CHAPTER 4

DIFFERENT WAYS OF FASTING

There are numerous known ways of fasting and they all offer the same benefits. These include healing, weight loss, cleansing and detoxification among others. The different ways of fasting are determined by personal preferences, reasons for fasting, any underlying issues and so on. Here is a look at different ways of fasting.

Intermittent fasting

The term intermittent fasting refers to a pattern where there is a period of eating and a period of fasting. It is a cyclic process with periods of fasting being longer than the eating periods.

It is very popular in the world today because of the benefits it is known for. Not only does it help improve your lifestyle but also your health and wellbeing and weight loss. It also has powerful effects on your brain and body and may enable you to live longer.

3 common methods of intermittent fasting

Eat-stop-eat method: In this method of fasting, you will fast for a period of 24 hours once or two times a week. You may choose not to eat any food once you finish dinner one day until dinner time the following day.

The 16/8 method: With this intermittent method, you rest for 16 hours and restrict your eating time to 8 hours. For instance, you may skip breakfast, have lunch at 12.00 noon and then dinner before 8.00 pm.

The 5/2 method: This is yet another form of intermittent. Under this method, you choose two days of the week when you eat only 500-600 calories and then eat normally on other days. These 2 days should not be consecutive.

Alternate day fasting

Another well-known fasting method is the alternate day fasting or AFD. It is a form of intermittent fasting where you eat what you want when not fasting but then you fast on every other day.
There are different forms of ADF fasting. These are known as modified forms of alternate day fasting. On one of these days, you may also choose to eat only 500 calories on your fast days which is equivalent to about 25% of your energy needs.

ADF fasting is a very effective form of weight loss. Adults who use this form of fasting often record a 3 – 8% weight loss within a period of 2 to 8 weeks. It is interesting to note that Alternative-Day Fasting seems to be more effective among middle-aged people compared to other groups.

Extended fasting

These types of fasting are also known as long-term fasts. The main purpose of long-term or extend fasts is weight loss. Basically, when you are not eating at all, you tend to lose weight pretty fast. These, on average, last about 4 days.

Some people consider extended fasts as dangerous. Others love them for their effectiveness. People trying to lose weight often hope that ketosis will kick in. this is when the body starts burning stored fat to produce the energy it needs. This is a great way to lose weight.

Another benefit of long-term fasting is cleansing. Extended fasting helps cells to cleanse themselves of toxins and other unwanted junk. This is because the cells have turned to consuming stored fats and are likely therefore to get rid of all other junk they come across.

People who fast continuously for a period of 10 days or so are likely to see benefits if they have hypertension. Many lose weight even though they had not set out to lose weight in the first place.

Weight loss definitely benefits anyone with hypertension or high blood pressure.

However, long-term extended fasting can be dangerous to your health. It may lead to starvation and eventual death. It is advisable to take a couple of things into consideration including contacting a medical doctor before embarking on a long or extended fast.

CHAPTER 5

WHAT TO EXPECT WHEN YOU START FASTING

Fasting has been around and is nothing new. However, people are taking to fasting lately because of the numerous benefits they can get. It is important to prepare yourself mentally and psychologically before embarking on a fast.

There are different stages of fasting and you should expect different experiences at each stage. If you know what to expect, then you can prepare yourself mentally and the experience will definitely help you along the way.

Hunger

In the initial days of your fast, you can expect to feel hungry. Your body is used to receiving nourishment on a regular basis and when this does not happen as expected then hunger pangs will set in. If you are mentally strong and psychologically prepared, then you should be able to overcome or withstand these feelings.

Reduction in energy

You are also likely to feel weak, suffering from a reduction of energy. While you are normally strong and in control, once you start fasting, you will very likely feel quite weak. Fortunately, this only happens at the begin but after a while, your body will get used to it.

Mood change and irritability

You are also likely to become very moody and irritable. Prepare yourself mentally for this phase because your patience will likely run out very fast. In the initial stages of fasting, your body will get into battery saving mode. Your blood pressure will drop and so will the heart rate. Your base metabolic rate will also adjust, becoming efficient and using less energy.

The first few days are, therefore, some of the toughest and you will feel like quitting. However, if you hang in there just a little longer, then you will very likely see a reduction in the severity of these symptoms. You will also benefit from the mental and physical challenges that you endure.

Cleansing and detoxification

Even as you continue to feel the hunger pangs, a lot of great things are happening to your body. Just knowing this can provide you with the psychological boost you need to withstand the challenges brought on by the fast.

As your body starts to react to the lack of food, it starts an internal process that will see most toxins eliminated. Also eliminated are dead cells, free radicals, and all unwanted matter. The cells are also likely to regenerate, creating new cells that are healthy, more effective and even efficient.

More energetic, less hungry

After a day or two, you will start to feel more energetic. At this stage, something call ketosis will kick in. This is when the body begins to burn fat stored in the body in order to provide energy. This will help you stop feeling tired or hungry.

It is important to note that ketosis does not need to happen only during a fast. You can start ketosis in your body by simply eating the right diet which consists of all the right kinds of food. You may want to learn more about what a ketosis diet is.

A clear head

Later on, if you proceed with your fast, you will get a clear head. Not only that but also your mood and temperament will improve drastically. By this stage, your body is beginning the healing process. This process begins with the digestive system. You will have very few free radicals in your body which then gets blessed with renewed cells.

Your blood sugar levels will decrease and then your pancreas will secrete hormones that will begin the process of converting the fat in your body into glucose. This can happen to either fat or protein within your body and will mark the beginning of your weight loss process.

You will finally break the fast and resume eating regularly. At this point, you should celebrate your achievement whether you fasted for half a day, an entire day or even a whole month. The benefits of the fast will become evident within a couple of days and will last a long time.

CHAPTER 6

HOW TO TRACK PROGRESS WHEN FASTING

Even as you fast, you should keep a track of changes that are happening to you and to monitor and note the progress that you are making. You may wonder about the best way to track progress during fasting. Jumping on a weighing scale may be tempting but on its own, it may be insufficient. This is because your body weight may vary from day to day by up to 2kg. There are a couple of other things you could do as well. Here is a look at some of them.

Tracking progress during fasting

1: Take waist measurements

If you are trying to lose weight, you should take measurements around your waist. For anyone who is losing weight for health reasons, then losing the fat around your waist is important. Take these measurements regularly and notice how frequently they change. A reduction means your health is faring well and you are losing the kind of fat that is dangerous to your body.

2: Weigh yourself every day (or almost) and average the figures

Most people weigh themselves, on average, every week. They do this in the bathroom using the home scales. However, if you are fasting, then you should start taking weight measurements almost every day. This is the best way of monitoring progress even as you fast.

Weighing yourself only once a week will not reveal the true story about your personal progress. This is because the amount of water your body holds varies. When you lose glycogen, you lose a lot more water. The same happens to the food you consume regularly. This food, contained in the body, will cause your body weight to vary significantly so daily weight measurement is a much better way of tracking your regular fasting as compared to weekly.

3: Weigh yourself on a monthly basis

You may alternatively choose to weigh yourself on a monthly basis rather than daily, weekly or almost daily. This is because you may achieve your weight loss goals within a month. If not, then you may lose a significant amount of weight in a month.

A few things you need to know is that weight fluctuates a lot so if you note changes, then you should not panic. Weight fluctuation is very normal. Another thing you should do is weigh yourself regularly, preferably on a daily basis and then plot these down on a graph. You will notice a trend which is a good indicator of your performance.

You should also measure yourself at the same time each time. For instance, if you weigh yourself in the morning after you wake up, then make this a habit and only weigh yourself at this time. This kind of consistency will reveal to you more accurate results compared to different weighing times.

4: Check your body fat levels

When people are trying to lose weight, what they really are trying to do is to lose body fat. It is significant, therefore, to also endeavor to measure how much body fat you are losing even as you fast.

In checking your body fat levels, you can use a body fat analyzer, usually found on weighing scales and sometimes just on their own. While they may not be very accurate, the body fat analyzers will provide you with an indication of the progress you are making.

This fat analyzer works by detecting the speed at which electric pulses takes to pass through your body. It will show you if your body fat is increasing or decreasing.

5: Blood pressure

You should check your blood pressure regularly. If you have high blood pressure, then a slight decrease in body weight can help lower your blood pressure. But remember, measuring blood pressure at different times of the day can result in different readings. It all depends on your state of mind as well as activity.

6: Blood glucose levels

Blood glucose levels are also a good indicator of your progress as you fast. One of the most prominent indicators of diabetes risk is high blood sugar. If you can keep this figure down, then you are doing great. There is a gadget that you can buy at the pharmacist to help you monitor your blood sugar levels.

CHAPTER 7

WEIGHT LOSS EFFECTS

One of the main reasons people choose to fast is to lose weight. Losing weight is great but it has many effects on your body. Weight loss also does a lot for you. It means more than just having an excuse to buy new clothes. There are some obvious and some not-so-obvious benefits. It is important to find out more about the benefits and effects of weight loss for motivational purposes and for general knowledge.

Obvious benefits of weight loss

When you lose weight, you feel great and also look great physically. A leaner frame and body enables you to be flexible and more mobile. Your movements are easier and accomplishing tasks becomes really easy.

When you look good, you also feel good. This helps boost your self-esteem and confidence. When your self-esteem is high, you will be confident enough to take on challenges, move up the ladder and be successful.

Your health gets better when you lose weight. For instance, you reduce the risk of getting conditions such as heart diseases, diabetes, and high blood pressure. Your overall health and wellbeing will also improve drastically.

When you lose weight, you will sleep better and experience improved moods. This can happen within the first couple of weeks and results from sleeping better and longer at night. Apparently, when you lose weight you tend to sleep much better. You are likely to experience increased mental focus during the fast. The reason is because your body releases chemicals into your body called catecholamines. These chemicals will result in increased productivity and alertness.

You will save money because you will buy less food and spend less on energy. Other obvious benefits include reduction of inflammation, a reduced risk of cancer, increased metabolism as you fast and burning off more of the stubborn fat, especially that around the midriff.

Less-obvious effects of weight loss Your memory levels will get better Studies have shown that when you lose weight, your brain will function better because your body sheds off plenty of toxins that made it hard for the brain to function at optimum levels

Energy levels will increase rapidly

People who lose weight often notice a significant amount of energy boost. When you carry around extra weight, you spend more energy carrying this weight around and less energy to do other things. When the weight is no longer on you, then you will have a lot more energy to spare.

You sleep better

It is a fact that when you lose weight you sleep better. According to research studies, if you lose 5% of your bodyweight, you will sleep better and for longer. When you shed pounds, you also avoid snoring and conditions such as sleep apnea.

You are likely to have a better mood

By fasting and losing weight, you will lose a lot of the toxins that clogged your mind and your body. The brain will also release a lot more of the feel-good enzymes such as endorphins. These will make you happier and have a better mood.

Less joint pain

When you carry excess body weight, your joints are likely to suffer due to the weight. However, by losing weight, you will suffer less joint pain. Even if you suffer from a condition affecting your joints, you will fare better if you lose weight.

Stress relief

Losing weight is one great way of relieving stress. We are all exposed to stress every single day. It is important to take measures to relieve stress and weight loss is a great way to achieve this.

Losing weight has plenty of benefits, some which are obvious and others not so obvious. Intermittent fasting provides an easy way to fast and lose weight in a healthy and sustainable manner.

Intermittent fasting is much easier compared to dieting

A lot of diets fail and the reason is because most of us are unable to stick with one over the long run. We tend to give up because the problem is not nutrition but behavior change.

It is much easier to try intermittent fasting because it is a much simpler concept to implement compared to dieting. It is also more effective when it comes to losing weight.

CHAPTER 8

HOW TO WARD OFF POTENTIAL NEGATIVE EFFECTS OF FASTING

Fasting is never an easy task, especially for a first-timer. You need to focus, get the right motivation and have goals in mind. If you can keep your mind on the goals you intend to achieve and the benefits of what you are embarking on, then you will be off to a great start.

You need to take each hour and each day at a time. Therefore, focus on small gains and celebrate each tiny milestone. If you focus on your entire fast, you may lose your motivation, especially if you set very high goals. There will be many tiny successes so ensure you savor each and every one of these. It is the small and gradual steps that will eventually enable you to achieve your bigger goals.

Intermittent fasting and other forms of fasting have such great benefits that sometimes it is possible to forget to be on the lookout for any negative effects. Like with all good things, there are some negatives as well. Here are some important steps you could take.

1: Do not indulge 100% because of initial low energy levels

When fasting, especially at the start, your energy levels are likely to be low. Therefore, do not expect to be full of energy like you usually are. Instead, rest more and avoid strenuous activity at least until you feel better. This is important because low energy levels can make you feel weak and possibly nauseous. Therefore, take precautions especially if you have to work or spend time engaging in intense physical or mental activity.

2: Watch your moods

Even as you fast, your moods are likely to change and you will most likely be grumpy and moody. You will snap at people, feel lethargic and have a generally negative attitude towards everything and everyone. Unless you are on a dry fast, then you may take a cup of coffee which will clear your mind. Fortunately, with time, you will be in great moods because fasting results in weight loss which means better sleep at night

3: You may suffer diarrhea or constipation

As you fast, you may suffer from either constipation or diarrhea. These are common during fasting. If constipation persists, then drink more water and take some apple cider. Also, add more fiber to your diet to ward off diarrhea episodes.

4: Binge eating

Binge eating is a real issue and very common once you break your fast. Gorging feels natural and people tend to overeat even after fasting diligently for a significant period of time. What you need is mindful eating and self-control. If you are disciplined enough to fast to the end, then you should be able to hold off the bingeing.

5: Fatigue caused by fasting

A lot of the time when fasting, we are also going to work and doing other regular activities. But if you are working out for long hours, working too hard at your job or having a negative talk, then all these will drain the little energy that you have. You should reduce your pace, relax and take things easy. Otherwise, you will burn out fast so learn to take life easy as you fast.

Intermittent fasting may not be so easy at first. Even seasoned individuals who have been fasting for years still face some of these challenges. Fasting has many great benefits for your body, mind and overall well-being. It is best to focus on the positives and use these to motivate you even as you face the negative side effects.

CONCLUSION

Thank for making it through to the end of this book, let's hope it was informative and able to provide you with all of the tools you need to achieve your goals whatever they may be.

Fasting is very important for your health and well-being. It will help you overcome many challenges that we encounter in our daily lives. But you should not just fast blindly. Find a good fasting plan that works for you then work around it until you are completely happy.

Remember that fasting is never easy and you will encounter many challenges. They range from hunger pangs, irritability, temptations, a lack of energy and so on. However, even at these moments, you should hold out and hang in there. Nothing good is ever easy and for you to enjoy the benefits you have to put in the effort.

First, come up with a good plan, start slowly and celebrate each and every tiny milestone. Always remember that others have made it through more rigorous fasts so you can too. Believe in yourself and you will eventually succeed.

Finally, if you found this book useful in any way, a review on Amazon is always appreciated!

** Remember to use your link to claim your 3 FREE Cookbooks on Health, Fitness & Dieting Instantly

https://bit.ly/2OazEZu

Printed in Great Britain
by Amazon